The Impact of State Voting Processes in the 2020 Election

Estimating the Effects on Voter Turnout, Voting
Method, and the Spread of COVID-19

SAMUEL ABSHER, JENNIFER KAVANAGH

For more information on this publication, visit **www.rand.org/t/RRA112-25**.

About RAND

The RAND Corporation is a research organization that develops solutions to public policy challenges to help make communities throughout the world safer and more secure, healthier and more prosperous. RAND is nonprofit, nonpartisan, and committed to the public interest. To learn more about RAND, visit www.rand.org.

Research Integrity

Our mission to help improve policy and decisionmaking through research and analysis is enabled through our core values of quality and objectivity and our unwavering commitment to the highest level of integrity and ethical behavior. To help ensure our research and analysis are rigorous, objective, and nonpartisan, we subject our research publications to a robust and exacting quality-assurance process; avoid both the appearance and reality of financial and other conflicts of interest through staff training, project screening, and a policy of mandatory disclosure; and pursue transparency in our research engagements through our commitment to the open publication of our research findings and recommendations, disclosure of the source of funding of published research, and policies to ensure intellectual independence. For more information, visit www.rand.org/about/research-integrity.

RAND's publications do not necessarily reflect the opinions of its research clients and sponsors.

Published by the RAND Corporation, Santa Monica, Calif.
© 2023 RAND Corporation
RAND® is a registered trademark.

Library of Congress Cataloging-in-Publication Data is available for this publication.
ISBN: 978-1-9774-1027-6

Cover: LeoPatrizi/Getty Images.

About This Report

This report is part of RAND's Countering Truth Decay initiative, which is focused on restoring the role of facts, data, and analysis in U.S. political and civil discourse and the policymaking process. The original report, *Truth Decay: An Initial Exploration of the Diminishing Role of Facts and Analysis in American Public Life*, laid out a research agenda for studying and developing solutions to the Truth Decay challenge. Truth Decay worsens when individuals lose trust in institutions that could serve as sources of factual information.

Funding

Funding for this research was provided by gifts from RAND supporters and income from operations.

Acknowledgments

We are indebted to Russell Hanson for his preparation of the SafeGraph weekly patterns data. We would like to thank the Center for Public Integrity for their generosity in sharing their polling locations data before their public release. Lastly, thanks to Ben Gibson and Daniel Thompson for thoughtfully reviewing this document and providing valuable feedback. Any remaining errors are ours alone.

Summary

Leading up to the 2020 general election, state election boards grew concerned that the coronavirus disease 2019 (COVID-19) pandemic might drive voters away from the polls or that crowded polling stations would spread the virus and lead to a wave of new cases, hospitalizations, and deaths. In an effort to safely conduct the election, many states changed their voting laws by implementing automatic voter registration, removing excuse requirements for absentee ballots, and expanding early voting windows. These changes, meant to encourage turnout and protect public health, were expensive to implement, politically contentious, or both. But did the changes have the desired effects?

   This report examines the impact of voting laws on voter turnout and choice of voting method (referred to from here on as *voting method*) in the 2020 election and the effects of in-person voting on the spread of COVID-19. However, it does not directly estimate the effect of state election processes on the transmission of COVID-19 during and following the 2020 presidential election. Below, we describe the relationships between voting laws and in-person voting on Election Day, and those between in-person voting and COVID-19 transmission.

   Although voting laws and their effects on voters' behaviors have long been an area of study for social scientists, the COVID-19 pandemic introduced additional risks to in-person voting and might have made flexible voting options, such as absentee ballots, more appealing to would-be voters. Throughout the report, we use an index to measure states' aggregate election flexibility that was created in a previously published RAND report, *An Assessment of State Voting Processes: Preparing for Elections During a Pandemic* (Kavanagh et al., 2020). The RAND flexibility index documents states' election processes and summarizes their flexibility along three dimensions: voting registration, early voting, and remote voting. States' election flexibility is rated as one of four scores: very low, low, medium, or high, which we use as the main measure in our analyses. Because the prior report rated states' election flexibility as of July 2020 and many states changed their voting laws between July and November 2020, we update states' election flexibility ratings for the November 2020 election (see Chapter 2).

In Chapter 3, we summarize our analysis of how election processes affected voter turnout and the methods that voters used to cast their ballots. In addition to studying the relationship between states' election flexibility scores and voter turnout using descriptive statistics, in the primary analysis, we use a panel of county-level voter turnout and a two-way fixed effects model to estimate the difference in the effectiveness of flexible voting policies in 2020 relative to their importance in past elections.

We then test whether voting laws changed the methods that voters used to cast their ballots. If voting laws kept polls from becoming overcrowded on Election Day, they might benefit public health by mitigating the spread of COVID-19. We use data from Aristotle, a campaign finance and reporting firm, that includes information on voting method in 2020. Although the data are large and contain rich information about voters' characteristics (e.g., income, race/ethnicity), this information is only available for the 2020 presidential election—a feature that prohibits the use of panel data methods (e.g., two-way fixed effects) to identify the effects of voting laws. Instead, we construct an empirical model that controls for several important covariates (i.e., factors that influence voters' choice of voting method but are not of direct interest). Only under restrictive assumptions does the model produce estimates of the causal effect of election processes on voting method. Instead, it is best to interpret the findings as robust conditional correlations.

Chapter 4 summarizes our investigation into election flexibility and its impacts on the incidence of in-person voting on Election Day. To identify visits to polling stations, we use anonymized cell phone data and records of polling station locations from SafeGraph and the Center for Public Integrity, respectively. The data are a cross section, which again limits the statistical tools available to us. We incorporate several important covariates into our empirical model to estimate how states' election flexibility affects the number of long visits to polling stations on Election Day. Finally, in our test of in-person voting's effect on COVID-19 spread, we employ both difference-in-differences and event study regressions to measure the static and dynamic causal effects of in-person voting during the pandemic.

It is our hope that the empirical evidence presented in this report will help inform future debate and policy on voting laws by documenting the effects of various election policies during a public health crisis. This report does not assess the effect of flexible voting laws on the incidence of voter fraud or public perception of election integrity.[1]

Key Findings

Trends in Voting Processes

States relaxed their voting laws leading up to the election. Fifteen states implemented changes to their voting processes, which led to increases in their aggregate election flexibility score between the concluding research date from Kavanagh et al., 2020, and Election Day on November 3, 2020. Figure S.1 maps states' election flexibility scores on Election Day.

Voter Turnout

The flexibility of states' election processes on Election Day increased voter turnout. Residents in states with higher election flexibility scores were 0.9 percentage points more likely to cast a ballot in 2020 than were residents in states with marginally lower scores. The ease of acquiring absentee ballots likely explains the higher turnout: Voters were, on average, 20 percentage points more likely to mail in their ballot than voters in less-flexible states.

Voting Behaviors by Demographic

The responsiveness to voting laws varied by demographic. Democrats were more likely to vote and far more likely to vote by mail than Republicans when offered more-flexible election processes. Among all ethnic groups considered, Black voters were least responsive to changes in election processes. Although estimates suggest that Asian voters were 27 percent more likely to use an absentee ballot when their state's election flexibility score increases, Black voters were only about 15 percent more likely to do so. We suspect that distrust in the security/efficacy of absentee ballots might

---

[1] For an assessment of the access and integrity implications of different voting processes and policy options, see Hodgson et al., 2020.

FIGURE S.1

Flexibility for Pandemic Preparedness Across Dimensions as of November 3, 2020

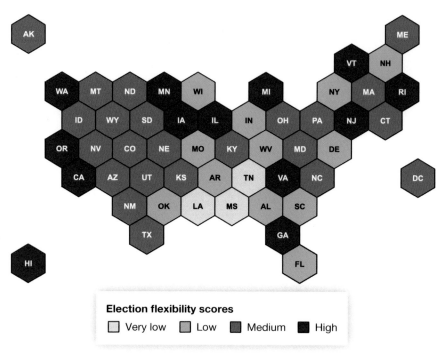

Election flexibility scores

Very low ☐ Low ☐ Medium ☐ High ☐

explain, to some degree, both Republicans' and Black voters' hesitancy to vote by mail, but we do not explicitly test this hypothesis.

In-Person Voting and COVID-19 Spread

States with less-flexible election processes had a larger share of their voters cast ballots in person on Election Day. This difference had consequences: U.S. counties with higher per capita in-person Election Day voting had higher rates of new COVID-19 cases in the first four weeks after the election. If America had completely eliminated in-person voting, our model predicts there would have been roughly 500,000 fewer new COVID-19 cases in the nine weeks following the election.

Conclusion

Taken together, we conclude that voting laws can mitigate the spread of COVID-19 and increase voter turnout by making remote voting more accessible. The results provide evidence of the importance of flexible voting laws—particularly for elections held during a pandemic.

However, this report is not a full cost-benefit analysis of election processes. We do not closely examine the financial costs that many laws and processes entail, or whether absentee ballots lead to greater incidence of voter fraud—though extant research shows voter fraud to be an exceptionally rare phenomenon, whether the ballot is cast in person or mailed in (Bump, 2016).

This caveat aside, the report does identify and, to the extent possible, quantifies three effects of flexible voting laws: (1) large increases in voter turnout, (2) reductions in in-person voting on Election Day, and (3) slower spread of COVID-19 in the weeks after the election. State legislatures should weigh these benefits as they assess the many proposals to change voting laws.

Contents

APPENDIX

Figures and Tables

Figures

Tables

CHAPTER 1

Introduction

The coronavirus disease 2019 (COVID-19) created unprecedented challenges for state election boards in the 2020 election. Although Americans typically cast their ballots in person on Election Day, in 2020, policymakers worried that the risk of COVID-19 exposure would deter voters or, alternatively, election day voters would crowd polling stations, potentially creating a wave of new COVID-19 cases. In an attempt to encourage voter turnout while maintaining election integrity and reducing the potential for COVID-19 exposure, many states changed their voter registration process, expanded early voting windows, removed barriers to absentee ballots, and made other changes to election policies and processes. But did these changes have the desired effects? In other words, what effect did changes in voting laws have on levels of voter turnout and, relatedly, what were the effects of in-person voting on the spread of COVID-19?

Economic theory suggests that voting laws affect would-be voters' behaviors. For example, theory suggests that restrictive voting laws impose nonfinancial costs to would-be voters and reduce their turnout (Riker and Ordeshook, 1968). It follows that, conversely, *more-flexible* election processes—including no-excuse requirements for absentee ballots, early voting, and automatic voter registration—ought to increase turnout by reducing voting's nonmonetary costs (e.g., time, need for transportation to the polls, concern about COVID-19 exposure). The theory of voters' responses to "costly" in-person voting has been validated in other settings. For instance, political scientists have shown that travel costs matter: When polling places relocate, voters who see their ballot box move farther away tend to use more-flexible methods (e.g., early voting) (Clinton et al., 2020).

Despite the plausibility of this theory, the research literature paints a complex and at times seemingly contradictory picture of the relationship between voting laws and would-be voter behavior. For instance, many suspect that laws requiring valid identification to vote burden voters and ostensibly reduce turnout—particularly among ethnic and racial minorities. But it has proven difficult to empirically identify an effect: Hajnal, Lajevardi, and Nielson (2017) argues that the implementation of strict voter identification laws reduces voter turnout, but Grimmer et al. (2018) shows that their findings are driven by data errors. A related study by Cantoni and Pons (2021) found no discernable effect, finding that states that implement such laws show similar rates of turnout and voter fraud. Similarly, intuition suggests that early voting and mail-in ballots, processes that offer flexibility to voters, should increase turnout, but the empirical evidence to date is also conflicted: A study of Ohio's 2010 homogenization law, which forced some counties to contract and others to expand their early voting periods, finds that voters in counties with longer early voting windows are in fact more likely to vote (Kaplan and Yuan, 2020); Burden et al. (2014) found that early voting in 2004 and 2008 national elections actually lowered turnout by reducing the civic significance of elections and made it more difficult for political campaigns to mobilize voters. These conflicting findings do not refute models of voters' behaviors per se but do highlight both the complexity and heterogeneity of voting laws' impacts and the challenges that researchers face when studying the effects of such policies.

Focus of This Report

This report attempts to shed light on these issues by quantifying the impact of voting laws on voter turnout and choice of voting method (referred to from here on as *voting method*) in the 2020 national election and the effects of in-person voting on the spread of COVID-19. Although voting laws and their effects on voters' behaviors have long been an area of study for both political scientists and economists, the COVID-19 pandemic allows us to study these processes when the costs of in-person voting are high and the potential benefits of flexible election processes ought to be most acutely felt by voters.

This report differs from earlier research because it studies the interaction between voting laws and the COVID-19 pandemic across the country.

We hypothesize that COVID-19 imposed a cost to in-person voting but that the magnitude of its effects will depend on each state's voting laws. However, there is nascent evidence that refutes this hypothesis: A recent study of voters in Texas and Indiana claims that removing excuse requirements for absentee ballots had little to no effect on voter turnout in 2020 (Yoder et al., 2021). Yoder et al. argues that when voters pay high costs to acquire information and care about its outcome, the costs posed by restrictive election processes are too trivial to drive voters from the polls.

Our work focuses on aggregate election flexibility rather than a single process or law and, where data permit, estimates its effects on all voters, not a single subset. We draw on an index created in a previously published RAND Corporation report, *An Assessment of State Voting Processes: Preparing for Elections During a Pandemic*, which documented states' election processes and summarized their flexibility along three dimensions: voting registration, early voting, and remote voting (Kavanagh et al., 2020). In the index, states received one of four scores: very low, low, medium, and high, which we use as the main measure in our analyses. Because the index rated states' election flexibility as of July 2020, and many states changed their voting laws between July and November 2020, we update states' election flexibility ratings for the 2020 general election.[1]

We then use this index and augment it with additional data to study the effect of aggregate election flexibility on voter turnout and voting method, with particular attention paid to its effect on the propensity of voters to cast their ballots in person on Election Day—the method that many feared would lead to a wave of new COVID-19 cases. To estimate the difference in the effectiveness of election flexibility in 2020 on voter turnout, we use county-level data on voter turnout from MIT's Election Data and Science Lab (MEDSL) and a two-way fixed effects (TWFE) model comparing turnout in counties with low election flexibility with those in states with greater election flexibility. We employ county- and election-level fixed effects because voting processes are not assigned randomly and differences in income, political preference, or education might influence the adoption of flexible voting process while also affecting voters' likelihood of casting a ballot. The

---

[1] The Cost of Voting Index also summarizes state voting processes into a single index. See Schraufnagel, Pomante, and Li, 2022, for additional information.

fixed effects model removes time-invariant heterogeneity (i.e., factors that remain fixed over time), and is commonly used to identify causal effects when a policy is implemented nonrandomly. We discuss its structure and the assumptions required for identification of causal effects in Chapter 3.

For our research on election processes' impact on voting method (i.e., early, remote, in person on Election Day) we acquire data from Aristotle, a campaign reporting and finance firm, that are available only for the 2020 election. Because we do not have data from earlier elections, we cannot use TWFE, a method that requires longitudinal data, and instead directly control for relevant confounding variables (i.e., race or ethnicity, political party affiliation, net worth, sex, and age). We also test whether voters of different racial or ethnic backgrounds (i.e., Asian, Black, Hispanic, and White) respond differently to election laws by choosing more-flexible voting methods by re-estimating the original model but restricting the data sample only to individuals belonging to that race or ethnicity. In addition to being prone to the same limitations (i.e., failure to identify the causal effect of state election flexibility), the analysis introduces an additional concern: A state's remote voting policy, one of the three dimensions in the RAND election flexibility index, theoretically has an outsized effect on voters' likelihood of voting by mail, but it holds equal weight in the aggregate index values. Thus, different racial or ethnic distributions across states with the same aggregate scores might actually have different remote voting laws—any findings of different effects across race or ethnicity might be attributed to their particular distribution across states rather than their responsiveness to flexible voting processes. This particular limitation is explained in greater detail in Chapter 3.

Next, we study the effects of election processes on the propensity to vote in person on Election Day in a county-level analysis. We identify visits to polling stations and estimate their duration using data on polling station locations from the Center for Public Integrity (CPI) and cell phone ping data from SafeGraph. Again, because we do not have data on previous elections, we cannot use empirical methods that require longitudinal data, so we estimate the effects of election processes on in-person Election Day voting by controlling for relevant covariates in our statistical model, including the share of Black residents, population density, the number of polls, and the number of Republican voters per capita.

Finally, we empirically test whether in-person voting exacerbated the spread of COVID-19. In this analysis, we use an event study design to show the effects of in-person per capita voting on new COVID-19 cases per capita over time. The event study model uses similar identifying variation and requires the same assumptions as the TWFE approach. There are limitations to this data. First, we only have access to polling location data for 37 of the 50 states. Second, not all SafeGraph places of interest (POIs), which we use to measure in-person Election Day voting, are matched to polling locations. The latter limitation could induce *attenuation bias*, which means that estimates of the effects of in-person voting might be biased toward zero.

Our research did not assess the effect of election flexibility on election integrity. Hodgson et al. (2020) assesses the access and integrity implications of different voting processes and policy options. However, it is our hope that the empirical evidence presented in this report will help inform future discussion and policy on voting laws by documenting any benefits shown to be associated with certain policies.

Organization of This Report

The remainder of this report is organized as follows:

- Chapter 2 describes the election flexibility index, explains the methodology behind the index's creation, and summarizes pre-election changes to voting laws.
- Chapter 3 presents the analysis of the relationship between the flexibility of states' election processes and voter turnout, focusing first on voter turnout and then on voting method. We also examine voting methods used by political party affiliation and race/ethnicity.
- Chapter 4 describes more explicitly the ability of voting laws to mitigate the spread of COVID-19 on Election Day by reducing the rate of in-person voting.
- Chapter 5 presents our conclusions.
- The Appendix provides a detailed accounting of the data and statistical models used in Chapters 3 and 4.

CHAPTER 2

The Flexibility of State Election Policies

In this chapter, we discuss the state election policies used to create the election flexibility index, and we provide assessments of states' level of election flexibility as of November 2020.

As described in Kavanagh et al. (2020), the index focuses on three dimensions of election flexibility: (1) voter registration, (2) early voting, and (3) remote voting. Table 2.1 lists more-flexible and less-flexible policies in each of the three dimensions.

In this chapter, we discuss these criteria in detail and explain any changes in states' election flexibility between July 2020, when Kavanagh et al. (2020) made their assessment, and November 2020, the date of our assessment. We then describe the rating system used and provide our assessment of state election flexibility scores as of November 2020.

State Election Processes in Place as of Election Day 2020

In this section, we discuss each dimension of the election flexibility index and summarize the changes that states made to their election processes before November 3, 2020. A more detailed discussion of these election processes can be found in Kavanagh et al. (2020).

TABLE 2.1

Three Dimensions of Election Preparedness During COVID-19 Conditions

Process	Less-Flexible Policies	More-Flexible Policies
Registration	• In-person registration • Advance registration	• Automatic voter registration (AVR) • Online registration • Same-day registration
Remote voting	• Excuse-required absentee • Early due dates for absentee ballots • Notary or witness signature required on ballot	• No-excuse absentee or mail-in option • Universal vote-by-mail • Later deadlines for absentee ballots • Witnesses not needed for voter verification
Early voting	• Early voting limited or prohibited	• Early voting (for extended periods)

SOURCE: Reproduced from Kavanagh et al., 2020, Table 1.1.

Registration

Voter registration is the first step that voters take to cast their ballot. As Kavanagh et al. (2020) points out, COVID-19 made registration more challenging for large swaths of would-be voters: Government buildings closed their doors, many people shied away from in-person contact, and election organizers canceled voter registration drives across the country. Before the election, the *New York Times* reported that COVID-19 led to drops in voter registration in several states (Wines, 2020).

Policymakers have at their disposal several tools to reduce face-to-face interactions in the registration process. One such solution is AVR. AVR combines voter registration with other in-person identification processes (e.g., getting a driver's license), thus eliminating the need for an additional face-to-face interaction to vote. Similarly, a second option, same-day registration, allows voters to register and cast their ballot during a single visit to the polling station on Election Day. A third option, online registration, eliminates the need for face-to-face contact entirely.

In theory, these policies can make it easier to register to vote during a pandemic; however, there are potential limitations to their effectiveness. Risk-averse voters might put off getting a driver's license during a pandemic, making AVR ineffective, while same-day registration could require an in-person trip to the polling station to vote. Online options are not equally available to all; for example, rural or poor voters might lack access to the internet or to the devices needed to register online.

Four states made changes to their voter registration processes before the 2020 election.[1] North Carolina made same-day registration possible during its early voting period, but not on Election Day (National Conference of State Legislatures, 2021). Similarly, Rhode Island allowed voters to same-day register, but only for the presidential and vice presidential race. Finally, a federal court ordered Virginia to extend its registration—from October 13, 2020, to October 15, 2020—after a fiber optic cable was accidentally clipped and took down the Department of Elections website.

Remote Voting

Remote voting received a significant amount of attention in the run-up to the 2020 election. On one hand, it was seen as a powerful tool to ensure access in a pandemic context that discourages people from congregating in person in large groups. On the other hand, some people raised concerns about the security of mail-in votes (e.g., whether they might be submitted by someone other than the registered voter).

Kavanagh et al. (2020) identifies several types of remote voting, which can be ordered from most to least restrictive: excuse-required absentee voting, no-excuse absentee voting, permanent vote-by-mail (in which an individual chooses to always vote by mail), and universal vote-by-mail (in which nearly all voting occurs by mail).[2] Even before 2020, most states had some sort of remote voting processes, though many states allowed remote voting only when voters met restrictive requirements.

Other areas of potential flexibility for remote voting include extending the deadline for receipt or postmark of absentee ballots and making changes to the verification processes used to ensure that the ballots received are legit-

---

[1]   A fifth, Maine, implemented automatic voter registration in 2022.

[2]   There is little evidence that remote voting contributes to increases in voter fraud. Confirmed cases of such fraud are rare.

imate (e.g., match to a signature on file, witness or proof-of-identification requirement).

Given the potential for remote voting to reduce virus transmission, it is little surprise that many (28) states adjusted their remote voting processes, making absentee ballots more accessible or extending submission deadlines. For example, such states as Alabama and Massachusetts no longer required excuses to use absentee ballots—perhaps the largest barrier to absentee ballots. Some states extended their postmark and receipt dates for mail-in ballots. Other states, such as Virginia, Alaska, and Minnesota, suspended witness or notary requirements for their remote voting processes. These changes were permanent for some states and temporary for others.

Changes to Remote Voting Policies and Processes Between July and November 2020

Figure 2.1 maps each state, highlighting those that underwent changes to their remote voting practices.

Among those states that did not change their voting policies, some already allowed universal vote-by-mail or no-excuse remote voting options, while others retained policies that limited remote voting options during the 2020 election. Kavanagh et al. (2020) offers more detail on which states fall into which category.

Early Voting

Early voting spreads polling station visits out across days or weeks instead of concentrating them in a single day, leading to shorter lines and less crowding. Early voting was particularly useful in the lead-up to the November 2020 election, when virus transmission at polling locations was a chief concern. Before 2020, most states permitted early voting, though its duration varied substantially, from 45 days to less than a week (Kavanagh et al., 2020). A handful of states set only a minimum period for early voting and allowed counties to expand early voting timelines at their discretion—in those cases, we used the state-level guidance to determine their early voting scores.

FIGURE 2.1

Summarizing Changes to Remote Voting Laws, July 2020 to November 2020

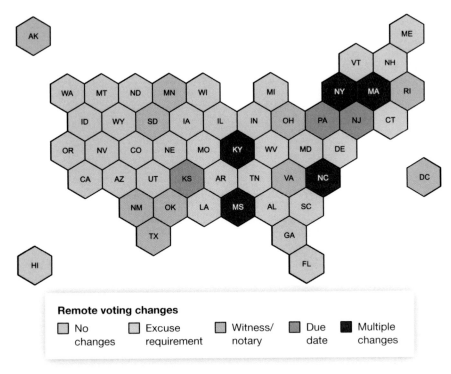

Remote voting changes

☐ No changes ☐ Excuse requirement ☐ Witness/ notary ☐ Due date ■ Multiple changes

SOURCE: State election websites and Ballotpedia, undated.

NOTE: Light tan indicates that a state underwent changes to their excuse requirement policy. Dark tan indicates that a state removed notary or witness requirements. Orange indicates that a state extended its submission deadlines. Red indicates that a state made multiple changes to its remote voting processes. Gray indicates that a state did not change its remote voting policies. See Kavanaugh et al. (2020) for a full review of the data collection methodology. Washington, D.C. is included in the voting flexibility index.

Changes to Early Voting Processes and Policies Between July and November 2020

As of July 2020, five states did not offer any early voting options while six others required excuses. However, several states made changes to their processes ahead of the general election in November. The most common change was to simply extend the early voting window, as Maryland did when it opened polls for eight rather the normal five days ahead of the general election. Rhode Island added in-person early voting in 2020 while Pennsylvania implemented a unique early voting option that allowed voters to request and submit an absentee ballot a month and a half before Election Day (Lai, 2020). But not all states expanded their in-person early voting access: New Jersey actually removed its in-person option in favor of expanding the period in which voters could either mail or drop off mail ballots (O'Dea, 2020).

Figure 2.2 plots the distribution of early voting duration for all states in the 2020 general election. All but four states (Alabama, Connecticut, Delaware, and New Hampshire) offered some form of early voting and states opened their polls (or ballot drop-off locations) an average of 19 days before the election.

Election Flexibility Scores as of November 2020

We now use the criteria laid out in the previous section to provide our assessment of states' election flexibility in the November 2020 general election.

Scoring System

As explained in Kavanagh et al. (2020), states receive one point for each dimension in which the state has more-flexible policies for the November 2020 election. Flexibility in each dimension was scored as follows:

- registration: at least two more-flexible policies as shown in Table 2.1 (AVR, online registration, same-day registration)
- remote voting: at least two more-flexible policies as follows: availability of no-excuse vote-by-mail, absentee ballot due dates of postmark by Election Day, verification processes that do not require witnesses or notaries
- early voting: state must offer early voting for a period longer than 16 days before the election.

The state's scores across the three dimensions are totaled to get the state's total election flexibility score:

- very low flexibility: 0

FIGURE 2.2

The Distribution of States' Early Voting Windows as of November 2020

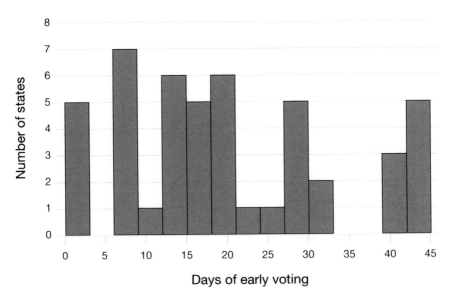

- low flexibility: 1
- medium flexibility: 2
- high flexibility: 3.

This measure of flexibility can also be seen as a measure of the resilience of the election process to other types of obstacles and disruptions to traditional election processes.

Kavanagh et al. (2020) assessed states' election flexibility as of July 27, 2020. Because many states made changes to their election processes after this date, we update that assessment in this report to account for policies in place as of November 3, 2020, the date of the national election.

Scores

Kavanagh et al. (2020) provided an assessment of state election flexibility scores as of July 2020. Using the above information on changes in states' election processes, we update the flexibility scores for the 2020 general election; these scores are shown in Figure 2.3. More detail on the coding methodology behind RAND's election flexibility scores can be found in Kavanagh et al. (2020).

Changes in States' Overall Election Flexibility Between July and November 2020

We also determined which states increased their election flexibility between July 2020 and November 2020. Figure 2.4 lists each state (and Washington, D.C.) according to the election flexibility score received in November 2020. The colors indicate whether the score changed from July 2020. States that increased their flexibility by one point are highlighted in blue; those that made two-point increases are in green.

The data show that states liberalized their election processes, easing restrictions on absentee and early voting. All 14 changes to RAND's elec-

FIGURE 2.3

State Election Flexibility Levels Across Dimensions as of November 2020

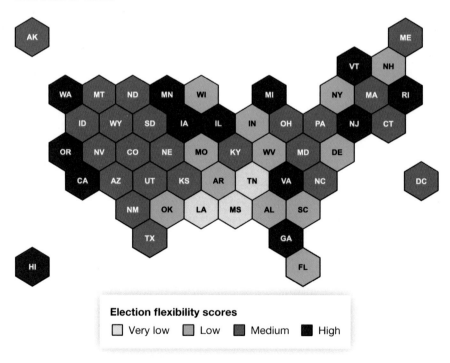

14

tion flexibility scores were increases—no state made their election processes less flexible leading up to the 2020 general election. Although these changes were made in response to the threat of COVID-19, they also might have had implications for turnout—who voted and how. We discuss this issue in Chapter 3.

Because of the coding methodology, states can change their policies without having aggregate changes in overall flexibility. Changes might appear instead in one individual dimension (e.g., early voting only or remote voting only) while not affecting relevant processes (i.e., automatic voter registra-

FIGURE 2.4

States' Election Flexibility Scores, November 2020, by Category and Change Since July 2020

Very Low	Low	Medium	High
Louisiana	Alabama	Alaska	California
Mississippi	Arkansas	Arizona	Georgia
Tennessee	Delaware	Colorado	Hawaii
	Florida	Connecticut	Illinois
	Indiana	District of Columbia	Iowa
	Missouri	Idaho	Michigan
	New Hampshire	Kansas	Minnesota
	New York	Kentucky	New Jersey
	Oklahoma	Maine	Oregon
	South Carolina	Maryland	Rhode Island
	West Virginia	Massachusetts	Vermont
	Wisconsin	Montana	Virginia
		Nebraska	Washington
		Nevada	
		New Mexico	
		North Carolina	
		North Dakota	
		Ohio	
		Pennsylvania	
		South Dakota	
		Texas	
		Utah	
		Wyoming	

Legend
- +0
- +1
- +2

NOTE: States that increased their election flexibility scores by one level are highlighted in blue. States that increased their scores by two levels are shown in green.

tion, no-excuse absentee ballots, and early voting availability) to increase the overall score.

Chapter Summary

In this report, we used an election flexibility index developed by Kavanagh et al. (2020). The index focuses on three dimensions of election flexibility: (1) voter registration, (2) early voting, and (3) remote voting. States receive one point for each dimension in which the state has more-flexible policies for the November 2020 election. States received points in each dimension as follows:

- registration: at least two more-flexible policies as shown in Table 2.1 (AVR, online registration, same-day registration)
- remote voting: at least two more-flexible policies as follows: availability of no-excuse vote-by-mail, absentee ballot due dates of postmark by Election Day, verification processes that do not require witnesses or notaries
- early voting: state must offer early voting for a period longer than 16 days before the election.

The state's scores across the three dimensions are totaled to get the state's total election flexibility score:

- very low flexibility: 0
- low flexibility: 1
- medium flexibility: 2
- high flexibility: 3.

We used the index to assess state election flexibility scores as of November 2020. We also indicated which states increased their election flexibility between July 2020 and November 2020. The data show that states liberalized their election processes, easing restrictions on absentee and early voting. All 14 changes to RAND's election flexibility scores were increases—no state made their election processes less flexible leading up to the 2020 general election.

CHAPTER 3

The Effects of State Election Processes on Voters' Behavior

As in other elections, Americans' decisions about whether and how to cast their ballots in 2020 rested on considerations of both the costs and benefits of voting. Though the ratification of the 24th Amendment made poll taxes illegal and removed voting's financial costs, voters still pay with their time and effort: Some voters must travel long distances to a polling station, and many face long lines once they arrive. But, for most Americans, voting's costs are outweighed by its benefits: concern for the election's outcome, a belief that their vote will influence it, or, perhaps, the thrill of civic engagement.

The year 2020 introduced an entirely new cost to in-person voting: the risk of COVID-19 exposure. Despite the pandemic, more than 66 percent of Americans (around 158.4 million) voted in the 2020 presidential election—an increase of roughly 5 percentage points from 2016. Turnout was high, in part, because voters were highly motivated: A Pew Research Center poll found that 83 percent of voters said it "really mattered" who won the election (DeSilver, 2021).

There is also suggestive evidence that states' election processes affected turnout. In a separate survey, Pew found that, of the 10 states with the largest increase in voter turnout from 2016 to 2020, seven conducted their election mostly, if not entirely, by mail. The Survey on the Performance of American Elections, an MIT poll that studies voters' experiences during the election process, estimated that 46 percent of voters used an absentee ballot in 2020, up from 21 percent in 2016 (Stewart, 2020). It is possible that an increased use of remote voting could be driven by concerns about COVID-19 exposure. A Harris poll found that more than two-thirds of Americans were "somewhat or very concerned" that they or their family members would be exposed to COVID-19 when visiting a polling station on Election Day (Cohut, 2020). In light of this, it would be far from surprising if voters preferred ballot drop boxes to polling stations in 2020.

Thus far, we have documented the landscape of U.S. state election policies, briefly discussed broad trends in voter turnout and voting method over time, and provided some suggestive evidence that election processes affected voters' behavior in 2020. With that background, we now turn to the main question we address in this chapter: "What were the effects of state election processes on voter turnout and voting method in 2020?"

We examine the effects of voting laws on turnout by (1) plotting changes in voter turnout from 2016 to 2020 by election flexibility index scores and (2) directly estimating the effect of states' election flexibility on turnout at the time of the election. The empirical model, which we will explain in greater detail, identifies not the effect of voting laws per se but the difference in the effectiveness of state flexible election processes in 2020 compared with their effects in 2012 and 2016.

How voters cast their ballots during a pandemic matters, too. In-person voting on Election Day might crowd polls and lead to the virus' spread. Thus, we test whether flexible voting laws reduced in-person voting on Election Day by allowing voters to use remote and early voting options. For this analysis, we use voter-level data from Aristotle, a campaign finance and reporting firm, and multivariable regression to estimate the effect of election flexibility scores on the propensity to vote (1) in person on Election Day, (2) in person early, and (3) by absentee or mail-in ballot.

Estimating the Effects of Flexible Election Processes in 2020

In this section, we explain the approach used to estimate the effects of election process flexibility on voter turnout in the 2020 election. We focus on the election policies and processes in place at the time of the November 3, 2020, election, regardless of when those policies were put in place.

Data Sources

To identify the difference in the effect of election processes in 2020 relative to past elections, we constructed an empirical model to explain voter turnout. The model allowed us to track counties' voting outcomes over time and test whether the availability of more-flexible voting options increased voter turnout in 2020 and whether the responsiveness differed by political party.

We acquired voting data from MEDSL. The data list each U.S. county's votes by candidate from 2000 to 2020. The data used in the model come from 3,110 counties or statistically equivalent areas (e.g., Louisiana's parishes) across three elections: 2012, 2016, and 2020, totaling 9,330 observations. We also used data from the U.S. Census' five-year American Community Survey (ACS) via the National Historical Geographic Information System's (NHGIS's) data portal. The ACS includes the total number of votes cast for each political party; the county's total population; the shares of the population that are White, Black, and Hispanic; and the county's median income. These data sources are summarized in Table 3.1.

We used these data to calculate the voter turnout (i.e., total votes for president divided by total population) and the Democratic and Republican voter turnout (i.e., votes for president *by candidate's political affiliation* divided by total population), both of which serve as outcome variables in our analyses. The data do not allow us to directly observe the votes by political party. We infer party by choice of candidate. For instance, if a registered Republican votes for Biden, their vote is recorded as a Democratic vote in our data.

TABLE 3.1

Summary of Data Sources Used

Source	Data Used in Model
MEDSL	• Data from 3,110 counties or statistically equivalent areas • Votes by candidate across elections in 2012, 2016, and 2020 • Total of 9,330 observations
ACS	• Each county's total population • Demographic information about race and ethnicity of population, median income

Two-Way Fixed Effects Analysis

To estimate the effect of election flexibility on voter turnout in 2020, we used what is known as a TWFE analysis, an extension of difference-in-differences. The TWFE technique uses longitudinal data (for this analysis, on county voter turnout across multiple elections: 2012, 2016, and 2020) to determine the effect of a specific treatment or policy (in this case, the level of election flexibility during the 2020 pandemic general election) on a specific outcome (i.e., voter turnout). However, our research differs from a standard TWFE model, which tracks treatment levels (i.e., election flexibility) over time. Instead, we observe only the election flexibility index in 2020, and our analysis implicitly assumes that states shared a common flexibility of 0 in previous presidential elections. In a sense, the treatment is not election flexibility per se, but the interaction of the COVID-19 pandemic and states' election flexibility score. The empirical model still informs the county fixed effect, by giving a sense of each county's typical voter turnout. This aspect of our analysis dictates the quantity we estimate in our empirical model. Rather than identifying the effects of election processes, as has been the objective of earlier academic studies, this strategy estimates how the effect of voting laws changed in the presence of COVID-19.

Pre-existing differences between different counties (e.g., in income, racial composition, education, age) make it difficult to parse the effect of a flexible election policy: Any measurable differences in voter turnout between counties could merely be the result of these pre-existing differences and not of the election flexibility policies. To address this challenge, TWFE accounts for time-invariant differences in voter turnout between counties that have policies with higher and lower flexibility before the policy is implemented and then compares that difference to the one that is measured after the policy takes effect. The difference between those differences (difference-in-differences) is the model's estimate of the policy's effect.

We illustrate the intuition behind TWFE using difference-in-differences as a motivating example. Although it differs from TWFE, it exploits similar identifying variation and its simplicity makes it better suited as an exemplar. First, let's assume that flexible election processes have **no** effect on voter turnout. Furthermore, let's say that high-flexibility states typically have higher voter turnout (e.g., 60 percent) than medium-flexibility states (e.g., 40 percent). In 2020, the pandemic and election processes change all voters' behaviors. Voters in high-flexibility states increase their turnout to 70 percent (+ 10 percentage points), while voters in medium flexibility states increase their turnout to 50 percent (+ 10 percentage points). A naïve comparison that looks only at the 2020 voting turnout by election flexibility category would suggest that flexible election processes increased voter turnout (70 – 50 = 20). However, the difference-in-differences estimate would rightly estimate that the flexible election processes had no effect on voter turnout, because the increase in high flexibility states (+ 10 percentage points) is no different from the increase of voter turnout in medium flexibility states (also + 10 percentage points).

In our analysis, the treatment at the center of the analysis is the flexibility of the state election processes in the 2020 election. We think of the 2016 and 2012 general elections as *pretreatment* observations—they help give us a sense of each county's business-as-usual voter turnout. We then assume that those differences would persist over time, which help us give a sense of how voter turnout would change in the absence of any differences in election processes. Any new differences that arise in 2020 between counties in the different election flexibility categories are attributed to the treatment. We provide a more-detailed description of the model and estimation strategy in the Appendix.

Effect of State Election Policies on Voter Turnout

Before discussing our estimates of the effect of state election policies on voter turnout, we note that voter turnout increased across the United States in the November 2020 election: There were approximately 136 million votes cast in the 2016 election but more than 158 million cast in 2020. Voter turnout increased in every state.

This increase is reflected in Figure 3.1, which plots each state's percentage change in voter turnout from the 2016 to the 2020 election. States are ordered first by election flexibility category (with the very low and low flexibility groups combined) and second by the size of their percentage change in turnout. By plotting the percentage changes in voter turnout from 2016 to 2020, the figure visually approximates the techniques employed in the model and its findings: Difference-in-differences uses the pretreatment

(2016) observations to get a sense of the expected differences between the groups. We calculate voter turnout for each year by the taking the total votes cast and dividing by the state's population in 2019.[1] We then measure its percentage change in voter turnout from 2016 to 2020 and plot it in Figure 3.1. States are sorted within their election flexibility category by the size of their percentage increase, from smallest to largest. The hollow diamonds indicate each group's average percentage increase in total voter turnout.

In addition to showing that voter turnout increased across the board, Figure 3.1 shows that there is a positive relationship between a state's election flexibility and its average increase in voter turnout. In other words, flexible voting practices do appear to have increased turnout. More-flexible processes appear to have accommodated risk-averse voters and created opportunities for new voters who might not have voted in previous elections.

States with less-flexible policies experienced smaller increases in turnout than states with highly flexible policies. High–election flexibility states saw an average increase of 17.42 percent in voter turnout, but states with low and very low flexibility saw jumps of 11.4 and 12.08 percent, respectively—an average increase of 11.54 percent between the two groups, which are plotted together in the figure below. States with medium flexibility fell shy of those with high flexibility but surpassed their peers that had very low and low flexibility, experiencing a 16.21 percent rise in voter turnout from 2016.

Although naïve comparisons between high- and low-flexibility states are unlikely to measure the true causal effect of state election processes on voter turnout, we estimate the parameters of two such cross-sectional models in 2016 and 2020, because these coefficients can help the reader understand and interpret the quantity estimated in the main empirical specification. Because the RAND election flexibility index was constructed just before the 2020 election and updated in this report to incorporate changes made in summer 2020, we use the original scores as proxies for the flexibility of state voting laws in 2016. The models employ the same county-level data that are

---

[1]   Although this is an imperfect estimate for the denominator (i.e., total number of eligible voters) that measure is not found in the ACS or MIT data. Its absence makes for less precise estimates, but it should not bias our estimates: States with higher election flexibility should not be any more or less likely to have unregistered voters in their population than the comparison groups.

FIGURE 3.1

Changes in States' Voter Turnout by Election Flexibility Score

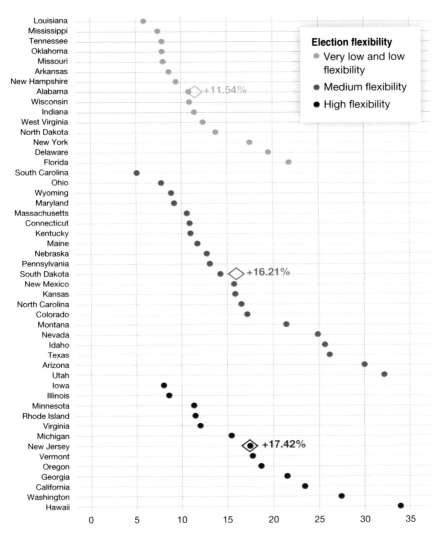

Percentage change in total voter turnout from 2016 to 2020 election

SOURCE: Features MEDSL's county presidential election returns data.

used in the primary model, but use only between-state variation to calculate the correlation between the flexibility of state voting laws and voter turnout. Finally, in a third model, we use the changes in state election flexibility scores to estimate their effect on voter turnout—the approach exploits variation only from the 15 states that liberalized their voting laws leading up to the 2020 election. The estimated coefficients of these regressions are found in Table 3.2.

In the 2016 model, we see that states with higher election flexibility scores (as proxied by their pre-2020 election values) have higher rates of voter turnout—though the differences are not statistically significant. A one-unit increase in a state's election flexibility score predicts a 0.3 percentage point increase in voter turnout. However, the 2020 effect is three times higher than the 2016 effect (0.9 percentage points). The difference between these two coefficients is the coefficient of interest in the primary model specification measures—i.e., the difference in the effectiveness of state election flexibility in 2020 relative to its effects in previous elections. These coefficients capture not only the states' election flexibility scores, but are also likely contaminated by a slew of omitted variables (e.g., income, political engagement, party affiliation), both observable and unobservable, that also explain why different residents of different counties have different propensities to vote in

TABLE 3.2

Cross-Sectional Comparisons and Changes in Election Flexibility

Coefficient Estimate	2016	2020	Change from 2016 to 2020
Election flexibility	0.003	0.009	−0.008
	(0.012)	(0.011)	(0.008)
Number of observations	3,110	3,110	6,220
R-squared	0.002	0.009	0.966

SOURCE: Features MEDSL's county-level presidential election returns data.
NOTE: The first two models (2016 and 2020) compare counties in states with varying election flexibility scores. The third model (labeled "Change from 2016 to 2020") measures how changes in the election flexibility scores affected voter turnout. Standard errors are clustered at the state level.

general elections. Thus, it is important not to interpret these results as the causal effect of flexible voting laws.

The final model (the column labeled "Change from 2016 to 2020") uses 2016 and 2020 data to estimate the effect of changes in state election flexibility on voter turnout between these two elections. The approach resembles that used in standard TWFE or difference-in-differences models, which use within-unit variation to estimate treatment effects. Here, we observe a negative and statistically insignificant coefficient estimate, suggesting that counties in the 15 states that liberalized their voting laws leading up to the 2020 election did not see measurable increases in their voter turnout rates.

We now turn to the primary empirical model and the estimates of its parameters. The findings suggest that, on average, a state moving up one election flexibility category (e.g., from very low to low, low to medium) increases its voter turnout by 0.9 percentage points in the 2020 general election. Though the effect is large in magnitude, it falls just shy of statistical significance in a 0.95 confidence interval. Its p-value, 0.058, lies above the 0.05 threshold that researchers often use to conclude an estimate is statistically significant, but it is close and falls under a more-flexible 0.1 threshold.[2] In other words, we find relatively strong evidence that flexible election processes increased voter turnout in 2020.

Although the county-level data do not describe votes by race or ethnicity, they do list votes for the Republican and Democratic candidates, allowing us to estimate the effect of election processes on voter turnout by political party. When we re-estimate its parameters, the model predicts that a one-unit increase in a state's election flexibility score increases Democrats' voter turnout by 1.2 percentage points on average. If all states had reduced their flexibility by one point, the model predicts that approximately 930,000 fewer votes would have been cast for Joe Biden.[3] Additionally, the estimate is strongly statistically significant—its p-value (0.00) is well below the standard 0.05 threshold. However, the effect on per-capita Republican turnout is statistically indistinguishable from zero. Democrats are more responsive to the availability of remote and early voting options than Republicans and

---

[2]   A p-value gives the probability that the estimated effect can be explained by chance (i.e., the effect is null and the estimate is not distinguishable from zero).

[3]   The calculation we use to arrive at this figure can be found in a box in the Appendix.

such policies do seem to confer benefits for Democrats more than Republicans, at least in 2020.[4] We propose explanations for these different responses in the following subsections.

Placebo Tests on 2012 and 2016 Elections

To validate the identification strategy employed above, we implement a pair of placebo tests that mimic the empirical methodology, estimating the effect of 2020 state election processes on voter turnout in the 2012 and 2016 presidential elections. If the identification strategy is sound, the exercise should uncover null effects of 2020's voting laws on 2012 and 2016. Both regressions use the same number of pre-treatment presidential elections (i.e., 2) and then estimate the effects of the 2020 state voting laws—the findings for the 2016 and 2012 placebos can be found in Table 3.3. In the six regressions we run, we find only one statistically significant estimate: the placebo test of Republican voter turnout in the 2016 presidential election. It is difficult to interpret how much this significant finding jeopardizes confidence in the primary analysis, but the null estimates found in five of the six (83.33 percent) tests is good. Placebo tests will wrongly return statistically significant estimates (i.e., a false positive) in some instances. The likelihood of false positives of placebo treatments depends on the bounds of the hypothesis test. Therefore, a 95 percent confidence interval has a 5 percent chance of a false positive, a 90 percent confidence interval has a 10 percent chance, and so on. Although the results cast some doubt on the method's ability to identify the causal effects of voting laws, particularly on voter turnout by political party, the placebo tests on all voter turnout is strong null in both instances. In fact, there is only one possible outcome in which we could have had more confidence in the empirical strategy we employ (i.e., zero statistically significant findings).

---

[4]   In 2020, much of the concern about the security and integrity of remote voting options was concentrated on the right side of the political spectrum, which might have affected the relationship between these provisions and turnout for Republicans.

Effect of State Election Processes on Voting Method

Aggregate election flexibility appears to have increased voter turnout in 2020 relative to 2016, but we know little of its effects on voting method, which has the potential to be consequential. Recall that the rapid liberalization of voting laws before the 2020 election was motivated by concerns that voters would crowd polls on Election Day and transmit the COVID-19 virus. The merits of election processes then lie in the extent to which they

TABLE 3.3

Placebo Tests of Election Flexibility Index

Panel A: 2012 Placebo Test			
Coefficient Estimate	All Votes	Democratic Votes	Republican Votes
Placebo effect	0.001	0.003	−0.002
	(0.004)	(0.002)	(0.003)
Number of observations	9,330	9,330	9,330
R-squared	0.960	0.968	0.971
Panel B: 2016 Placebo Test			
Coefficient Estimate	All Votes	Democratic Votes	Republican Votes
Placebo effect	0.001	0.004	−0.007*
	(0.003)	(0.004)	(0.003)
Number of observations	9,330	9,330	9,330
R-squared	0.967	0.956	0.969

SOURCE: Features MEDSL's county presidential election returns data.
NOTE: The parameters are estimated using an ordinary least squares regression (from the Stata command "reghdfe") with county and election fixed effects. In columns two and three, we use only the number of votes for the Democratic and Republican candidates, respectively. The coefficient of interest is election flexibility placebo which gives the effect of a one-unit increase in the election flexibility placebo on voter turnout. Panel A contains estimated placebo effects for the 2012 general election and Panel B the results for the 2016 placebo. * statistically significant result.

both improve voter turnout and protect public health by reducing polling station congestion.

To assess these processes' impact on the latter outcome, we first estimate the effects of election processes on voting method: Are voters in states with flexible election processes more likely to use remote and early voting options? For this section, we use National Consumer File (NCF) data, which come from Aristotle, a campaign finance and reporting firm. The NCF data are large and highly detailed, containing estimates of net worth, ethnicity, voting method, political party affiliation, state of residence, and age for more than 250 million Americans. We did not use the NCF data in the previous analysis because, although these data are more disaggregated (i.e., at the individual level) and contain additional voter information (e.g., net worth, ethnicity), the data only cover the 2020 election, which prohibits the use of difference-in-differences models that are able to identify causal effects under less-restrictive assumptions.

Figure 3.2 plots the percentage of voters who cast their ballots early, in person on Election Day, or remotely for all voters and for subgroups of voters based on their political preference and race or ethnicity. We find that 18 percent of all voters cast their ballots early and in person in the 2020 general election, 40 percent voted in person on Election Day, and 42 percent voted remotely.[5]

The second two rows in Figure 3.2 show the voting method distributions by political party registration, and the final four rows of this figure break down voting method by race or ethnicity. Registered Democrats were more likely to use absentee ballots (48 percent) than registered Republicans (36 percent), who tended to vote in person, either early (20 percent) or on Election Day (44 percent).[6] Confidence in the security and validity of absentee ballots might explain some fraction of this difference between political parties. According to a 2020 Pew Research poll, 43 percent of Republicans said voter fraud has been a major problem when it comes to voting by mail

---

[5] For reference, these figures are comparable to a 2020 Pew Research Poll, in which 46 percent of voters surveyed claimed to have used a mail-in ballot for the presidential election (Pew Research Center, "3. The Voting Experience in 2020,"2020b).

[6] *Democratic voters* and *Republican voters* refer to voters registered as Democrats and Republicans. Their votes for the presidential candidates are unknown.

FIGURE 3.2
Voting Method by Group

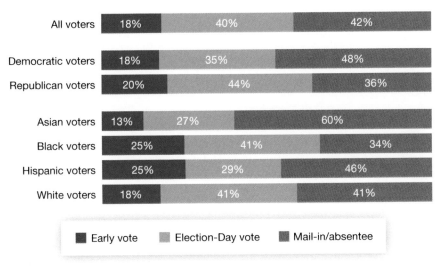

SOURCE: Features data from NCF.
NOTE: Percentages by political party indicate the share of registered Republicans or Democrats who used a particular voting method.

in U.S. presidential elections and another 31 percent said security of mail-in votes are at least a minor problem (Mitchell et al., 2020). Almost half of all Democrats surveyed felt that voting by mail was not prone to fraud. Democrats also expressed more concern about COVID-19 exposure and therefore might have been leery of polling stations. A July 2020 Pew survey found that 85 percent of Democrats considered the COVID-19 pandemic a major threat to the health of the U.S. population, while only 46 percent of Republicans did (Tyson, 2020). An earlier survey, taken in June, revealed that only 35 percent of Republicans were concerned that contracting COVID-19 would require hospitalization, compared with 64 percent of Democrats (Pew Research Center, 2020a). Among all included groups, Black voters were least likely to use mail-in ballots (34 percent), while Asian voters were the most likely to (60 percent).

Voting Method by Election Flexibility Score

In Figure 3.3, we plot voting method shares by election flexibility category. The descriptive statistics suggest that voters from states with a high

FIGURE 3.3

Voting Method by Election Flexibility Score

High flexibility	30%	70%	
Medium flexibility	31%	33%	36%
Low flexibility	16%	60%	24%
Very low flexibility	36%	62%	

■ Early vote　■ Election-Day vote　■ Mail-in/absentee

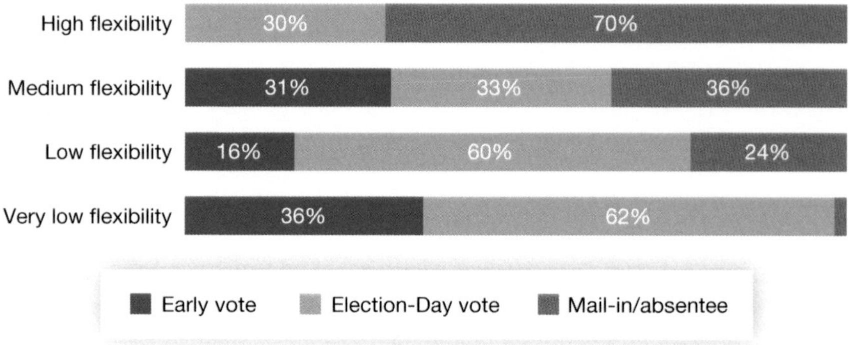

SOURCE: Features data from NCF.

flexibility score were far more likely to vote remotely than those in states with more-restrictive processes—about twice as likely as voters in the next most-flexible category, medium, and three times more than voters in low-flexibility states. Only 2 percent of voters in very low election flexibility states voted remotely in 2020. However, there is no clear relationship between election flexibility score and early voting.

Although this analysis reveals a strong correlation between states' election flexibility and voters' propensity to vote by mail, it does not demonstrate a causal relationship. In other words, although there is an association between a state's election flexibility and voters' decision to vote by mail, we do not know whether election flexibility caused that outcome. The problem of selection bias confounds any causal interpretation of the relationship; voters in states with more-flexible election laws tend to be wealthier and more liberal than voters in states with less-flexible processes, and they are likely different along other unobserved dimensions. Therefore, simple comparisons between voting methods across the election flexibility indexes, such as that pictured in Figure 3.1, fail to disentangle the effect of election processes from differences in voters' preferences, characteristics, resources, etc.

To address this problem, we constructed an empirical model to explain voters' selection of voting method. Voters in the model select one of four methods: (1) absentee, (2) in person on Election Day, (3) early in-person, and (4) not voting or abstention. The model's explanatory variables include controls for factors that we suspect also affect voters' decision (i.e., their race and ethnicity, political party, wealth, and age) and a variable for the election flexibility score of the voter's state. We estimate the parameters of the model using data from Aristotle's NCF and RAND's state-level election flexibility index.[7]

We find that the relationship between election flexibility scores and tendency to vote by mail persists. Voters in states with marginally higher election flexibility scores (e.g., voters in medium- compared with low-flexibility states) are on average about 21 percentage points more likely to vote by mail after controlling for the listed covariates. The large (and statistically significant) effect of election flexibility scores on voters' tendency to mail in their ballots is, to some degree, unsurprising. Remote voting, and specifically no-excuse-required absentee ballots, amounts to one-third of RAND's flexibility index calculation. It follows intuition that voters in states that remove excuse requirements or, alternatively, conduct their entire election by mail, are more likely to cast absentee ballots. However, we find no statistically significant effects of election flexibility on in-person voting. It is possible that voters switching to remote voting from the three remaining voting options (i.e., in person on Election Day, early in-person, or abstention) explains their statistical insignificance.

Furthermore, any analysis depends on the quality of the data used to estimate the model's parameters. But, because the Aristotle data are proprietary, little is known about the exact methodology used to gather information about voters' behaviors and characteristics, making it impossible to precisely identify or quantify the possible biases or limitations the data impose. For example, Aristotle relies on state agencies to report individual voting method, suggesting that data quality might vary by state, which could lead to reporting bias. If states with higher election flexibility are more likely to report remote or early votes than states with lower election flexibility, the analysis might wrongly indicate that voting laws increased voters' use of flexible voting options when, in fact, the finding is merely a result of reporting bias. For these reasons, we conduct an additional analysis that estimates

---

[7] Details about the data, model, and estimation can be found in the Appendix.

the relationship between voting laws and in-person voting on Election Day in Chapter 4.

Voting Method by Race or Ethnicity

Voting is not equally accessible to all Americans. Past research has shown that minority voters face longer polling lines on Election Day and suffer disproportionately from strict voter ID laws (Chen et al., 2020). Flexible election processes might allow voters to avoid long lines and, ultimately, improve turnout among demographics with perennially lower turnout. We test this hypothesis by measuring demographics' responsiveness to their state's election flexibility score by removing all individuals who do not fit the demographic criteria and using this subsample to re-estimate the model's parameters. The estimates tell us how the demographic in question responds to aggregate voting laws, but they are difficult to interpret in their raw form. Table 3.4 presents their average marginal effects on each voting method.

We find that Asian voters were most responsive to flexible election processes: An increase in a state's election flexibility score increases their likelihood of casting an absentee ballot by 27 percentage points. Black voters, on the other hand, were the least responsive. Increases in the state election flexibility index predict only a 16 percentage point increase in Black voters' use of absentee ballots. Their relative reluctance to vote by mail could be explained, in part, by institutional distrust (Williams, 2020). There is a history of suffering from policies aimed at deterring the Black vote. A Pro-

TABLE 3.4

The Effects of Election Flexibility Scores by Race or Ethnicity

Voting Method	Race or Ethnicity			
	Asian	Black	Hispanic	White
Absentee	27 percent	16 percent	19 percent	21 percent
Election Day	–11 percent	–10 percent	–5 percent	–10 percent
Early	–7 percent	–3 percent	–10 percent	–7 percent
Abstain	–10 percent	–3 percent	–4 percent	–4 percent

NOTE: The results listed here are interpreted from the raw estimates and presented in percentage points. The raw estimates can be found in the Appendix. Statistically significant findings are highlighted in gray.
SOURCE: Features NCF data.

Publica investigation of the 2018 midterms showed that absentee ballots from Black voters were far more likely to be rejected than mail-in votes from White voters (Chou and Dukes, 2020). For this reason, Black voters might feel more comfortable casting their votes in person (or abstaining), even if an absentee ballot is relatively accessible.

Another possible explanation for these results is that racial and ethnic groups are unevenly distributed across states with more- and less-flexible remote voting processes. To illustrate this alternative explanation, first recall that the RAND election flexibility index measures the flexibility of election processes across three dimensions: registration, early voting, and remote voting. Second, imagine three states, say A, B, and C, that have election flexibility scores of very low (0), low (1), and low (1), respectively. Say state B has inflexible remote and early voting processes (+0), but flexible voter registration (+1), and state C has flexible remote voting laws (+1) but inflexible early voting and voter registration processes (+0). Both states B and C receive the same election flexibility scores but impose different costs to remote voting. Third, assume Asian voters disproportionately live in state C (flexible remote voting), while Black voters tend to live in state B (flexible voter registration). The empirical model compares the responsiveness of voters in state A to those in states B and C, which are grouped under the same election flexibility score of 1. The finding that Asian voters are more responsive to election flexibility might be driven by the fact that their change in election flexibility is disproportionately driven by their propensity to live in state C, where the costs to remote voting are lower, while Black voters compared across state A and states B and C tend not to see their costs of remote voting lowered, so their perceived responsiveness is lower. Given that the model does not dismiss this possibility, the interpretation that responsiveness to voting laws varies by race or ethnicity must be taken with some caution.

Chapter Summary

In this chapter, we estimated the effect of flexible voting laws on voter turnout and voting method. We found that flexible voting laws led to slightly higher voter turnout, but the biggest impact was on voting method: Voters in states with flexible voting laws were 20 percent more likely to vote by mail, suggesting that the use of this method reduced congestion at polls on Election Day.

These effects were not equally distributed: They varied by political affiliation and ethnicity. Registered Democrats were more responsive than registered Republicans to changes in voting laws: A one-unit increase in election process flexibility increased Democratic turnout by 1.2 percentage points, but we find no statistically significant effect on Republicans' turnout. Black voters were least responsive to changes in voting laws.

We provide some suggestive evidence that institutional trust moderates the efficacy of voting laws. Republican leaders repeatedly called into question the security of absentee ballots leading up to the election, and members of the party expressed concern about the use of absentee ballots. This messaging and Republicans' subsequent reluctance to vote by mail might explain their muted reaction to flexible election processes relative to the reaction by Democrats. Possibly concerned that their absentee ballots might not be counted, Black voters too preferred to cast their ballot in person more often than White, Asian, or Hispanic voters.

These findings provide suggestive evidence for the hypothesis that the efficacy of voting laws depends on the public's trust in institutions and subsequently their willingness to exploit them. To maximize their return on remote and early voting infrastructure, state election boards might benefit by further emphasizing the safety and security of these options.

CHAPTER 4

State Election Policy and COVID-19 Spread

Chapter 3 demonstrates that flexible election processes increased turnout in 2020 and greatly increased the use of remote voting. It also presents evidence that flexible voting processes lowered in-person voting on Election Day by increasing use of absentee ballots. But we know little about the extent to which the use of absentee ballots lowered congestion at the polls and whether crowded polls worsened the spread of COVID-19.

Existing research exploring Election Day voting and its effects on the pandemic is mixed. A recent study of Wisconsin's presidential primary election showed that a 10-percent increase in in-person voting was associated with an 18.4-percent increase in COVID-19 positive test rates two to three weeks later (Cotti et al., 2021). Another study comparing counties with similar population density, age, income, and Republican vote share in the 2016 election found that whether a county held a primary or not had no measurable effect on COVID-19 spread (Feltham et al., 2020). Research on in-person voting's effect on COVID-19 transmission during the general election has begun to emerge as well: A 2021 article from *The Economist* reported that counties in the highest quintile of in-person voting on Election Day saw eight more cases of COVID-19 per capita than their peers in the second quintile and four more than counties in the first (and lowest) quintile. The authors reason that if states had removed in-person voting and moved entirely to absentee ballots, as New Jersey did, there would be 220,000 fewer COVID-19 diagnoses after the election ("In-Person Voting Really Did Accelerate COVID-19's Spread in America," 2021).

In this chapter, we seek to answer two questions: First, did voting laws, as measured by RAND's election flexibility index, affect the incidence of in-person voting during the November 2020 election? Second, did in-person voting exacerbate the spread of COVID-19? The research design uses cell phone ping data from SafeGraph and polling location data from the CPI to identify confirmed visits to polling stations on Election Day. We begin this chapter by examining the effects of election processes on the incidence of in-person voting and describe the data in detail. We then estimate the costs that in-person voting imposes on the public in terms of new COVID-19 cases.

Estimating the Effect of State Election Processes on In-Person Voting

Estimating the effect of election processes on the incidence of in-person voting requires information on states' election processes, which RAND's election flexibility index measures, and data on the amount of in-person voting in a specific location (e.g., a U.S. county). To construct the latter measure, we first acquire data on polling locations across the country in the 2020 election. Each state gathers and stores its own polling location data. The CPI reached out to states to gather their Election Day polling location data for 2020 and shared their data with us before its public release. The CPI data cover 34 states and a total of 103,891 polling stations. Many states send the addresses of polling locations but not their latitude and longitude. CPI geolocates these addresses and successfully estimates longitude and latitude coordinates for 102,414 (98.6 percent).

Figure 4.1 plots polls that were successfully geolocated over a map of U.S. counties, which we downloaded from the Census Bureau. States that offered only vote-by-mail in the 2020 election (e.g., New Jersey) or simply did not provide data on polling locations are grayed out.

Table 4.1 summarizes the number of polling locations by state.

Next, we use the CPI data and SafeGraph's Weekly Patterns data to estimate the number and duration of Election-Day polling station visits. In its raw form, the Weekly Patterns data lists visits to more than 4.5 million POIs in the United States each week using information from cell phone pings. SafeGraph POIs include businesses, churches, hospitals, government buildings, and other locations across the United States. To identify a polling-

FIGURE 4.1

Election-Day Polling Locations in 2020

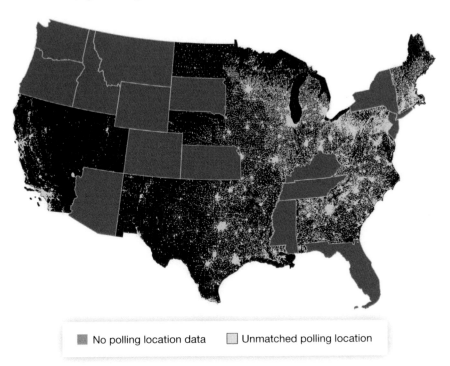

No polling location data   Unmatched polling location

SOURCE: Features CPI data.
NOTE: This figure maps each of the polling places from the CPI in the states where data are
available for the 2020 election.

station visit, we must first determine SafeGraph POIs that are polling locations. This is difficult. The polling station geolocation process is, in some
cases, imprecise and might only approximate a poll's location, which makes
automating the SafeGraph–poll matching procedure challenging. Given
the data's size, it is far too time-consuming to match the two manually. In
our preferred specification, similar to Chen et al. (2020), we match using
a 100-meter radius around each polling site. If a SafeGraph location falls
within this range, it is identified as a polling station.

Using the 100-meter radius rule, we successfully matched 68.3 percent of
CPI polls. Expanding the radius increases the number of successful matches

TABLE 4.1

Number of Polling Locations by State

State	Number of Polls	State	Number of Polls
Alaska	441	North Carolina	2,662
Alabama	2,075	North Dakota	858
Arkansas	967	Nebraska	982
California	3,853	New Hampshire	339
Connecticut	747	New Mexico	537
Delaware	434	Nevada	772
Florida	421	Ohio	8,933
Georgia	2,678	Oklahoma	1,938
Iowa	1,681	Pennsylvania	9,235
Illinois	10,013	Rhode Island	500
Indiana	1,964	South Carolina	2,302
Louisiana	3,934	Texas	7,556
Massachusetts	2,173	Utah	118
Maryland	321	Virginia	2,485
Maine	630	Vermont	261
Michigan	4,750	Wisconsin	7,092
Minnesota	4,110	West Virginia	1,729
Missouri	14,354	Total	103,845

SOURCE: Features CPI data.

but also increases the risk of false positives. Table 4.2 lists the different radii used and their respective match rates.

Figure 4.2 plots the polling stations from CPI and highlights in pink those that are successfully matched to SafeGraph POIs using the 100-meter matching radius. Unmatched polls are in yellow.

The Weekly Patterns data provide the number of weekly visits to Safe-Graph POIs and the number of visits by duration in minutes (i.e., less than 5,

TABLE 4.2
SafeGraph Location to Poll Match Rate by Search Radius

Distance (Meters)	Match Rate (%)
50	51.79
100	68.26
125	73.12
150	76.67
200	81.37
500	90.38

SOURCE: Features data from SafeGraph and CPI.
NOTE: *Match rate* is the number of successfully matched polling locations over the total number of polling locations.

between 5 and 20, 21 and 60, 61 and 240, and more than 240). It also lists the number of visits on a given day, but not their duration.

Figure 4.3 plots the visits to polling stations by duration each week over time. During the week of the election (November 3, 2020), we observe large increases in visits to locations identified as polls lasting between 5 and 20 minutes and those between 21 and 60 minutes; there is a smaller, but still visible, increase in visits between 61 and 240 minutes—findings which are consistent with descriptions of polling wait times in the 2020 election in other sources (Quealy and Parlapiano, 2021).

Not all visits to polling locations are made to cast votes—even on Election Day. Polling locations often serve other functions (e.g., schools, churches, offices), which means that individuals might visit for reasons unrelated to the election. To disentangle voting visits from nonvoting visits, we subtract the number of visits to the polling sites in the following week, which we consider a good indicator of the number of visits that would occur on November 3, 2020, had there been no election. Alternatively, we could use the preceding week as a counterfactual, but, in many cases, the Election-Day polling site serves as an early voting site too, which might bias the estimate of Election-Day voting visits.

FIGURE 4.2

Matched and Unmatched Election-Day Polling Locations in 2020

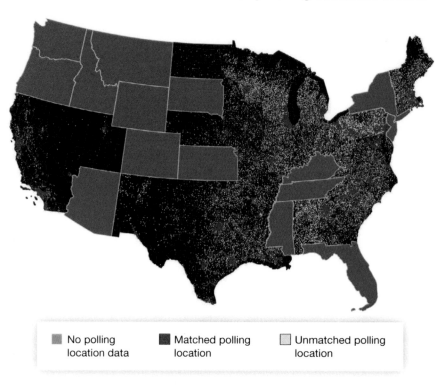

| | No polling location data | | Matched polling location | | Unmatched polling location |

SOURCE: Features data from SafeGraph and CPI.

Relationship of Election Flexibility and In-Person Polling Visits

Table 4.3 lists descriptive statistics by states' election flexibility score. Some interesting patterns emerge. Despite having more polling locations per capita, which we expect to reduce congestion, as measured by "visits per poll," we find that states with higher election flexibility had fewer visits to polling locations on Election Day. Louisiana, the sole very low flexibility state for which polling station data was available, had roughly 42 polls per 100,000 people. However, we identified 1,693 long visits per poll. In comparison, the nine states with high election flexibility had only 23 polls

FIGURE 4.3

Duration of Visits to Polling Stations Over Time

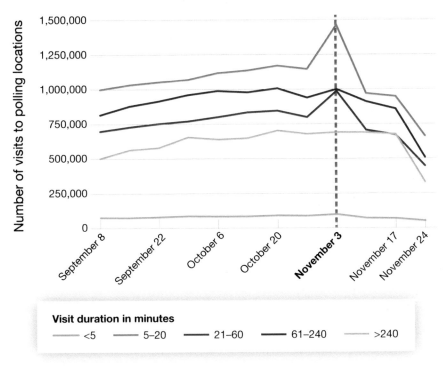

Visit duration in minutes

—— <5 —— 5–20 —— 21–60 —— 61–240 —— >240

TABLE 4.3

Election Processes, Population, and Polls

Flexibility Score	Number of States	Number of Polls	Population (in 100,000s)	Polls per 100,000	Long Visits per 100,000	Percentage Matched Polls
0	1	1,958	46.64	41.98	1,693.69	0.60
1	10	14,571	395.13	36.88	1,227.22	0.54
2	14	23,566	923.23	25.53	854.00	0.63
3	9	21,321	912.62	23.36	698.38	0.65
—	17	—	969.35	—	—	—

SOURCE: Features data from SafeGraph and CPI.
NOTE: Dashes indicate empty cells where no polling location data were available.

per 100,000 people, but only 698 visits per 100,000 people. The trends are consistent with the hypothesis that flexible voting laws reduced in-person voting. We test this relationship in greater depth later in this chapter.

For the model and the estimates of its parameters, we use county-level data that include the number of polling stations within the county, the number of visits by duration for Election Day (November 3, 2020), the total number of votes cast in the county, and the county's election flexibility score. The data cover 2,191 U.S. counties, each of which has an average of 28 polls. It identifies a total of 751,199 Election-Day polling station visits.

We are most interested in polling stations visits that exceed 15 minutes, because Centers for Disease Control and Prevention guidance defines an incidence of "COVID-19 exposure" as close contact (i.e., within 6 feet) with a carrier that lasts more than 15 minutes (Centers for Disease Control and Prevention, 2022). The SafeGraph data describe the duration in minutes of polling station visits in bins (e.g., less than 5, between 5 and 20, between 21 and 60) and, although the bins do not separate nicely on the 15-minute mark, they do allow us to identify and test for effects on longer visits. For this reason, we estimate the effect of states' election flexibility scores on the number of polling station visits per 100,000 votes cast that last between 20 minutes and four hours, which we call *long* visits.

The SafeGraph data cover only polling station visits for 2020, so we cannot see how polling station visits change from past elections based on election flexibility. Instead, we construct an empirical model that controls for important confounders, such as racial composition and income at the county level and compare the level of in-person voting across counties with different election flexibility measures. As we mention in our analysis of state election processes and their effect on voter turnout, creating a model that controls for all potential confounders is difficult if not impossible. For this reason, we note that estimates of parameters in the model could be affected by omitted variable bias and should be interpreted as conditional correlations rather than causal effects.[1]

---

[1] Models that use panel data (e.g., difference-in-differences, fixed effects) are not immune to omitted variable bias. But those models do control for all time invariant heterogeneity and require weaker assumptions to interpret findings as causal.

The model controls for several confounding variables. Areas with high minority populations often face longer wait times on Election Day—mostly because they have fewer polling stations per capita, and so we add controls for the share of the county's population that is Black and the number of polls per capita. Income and population density matter too: Voters in richer counties typically face shorter waits than those in poorer counties, while polling locations in populous areas tend to have longer lines on Election Day, so we include county-level measures of income per capita and population density from the NHGIS data portal (Manson et al., 2021; Weil et al., 2019). Republicans, as demonstrated earlier in this report, preferred to vote in person, so the county's share of Republican voters is included as a control. We then include the election flexibility score as a predictor variable and observe the correlation between it and the number of long visits to polling locations per 100,000 votes cast in the county (i.e., the predicted or *outcome* variable) that remains after controlling for the covariates. The reader can find a full description of the model and results in the Appendix.

We find that flexible election processes are negatively correlated with in-person votes per capita, even after controlling for the array of demographic and political variables we list above. In other words, states with lower election flexibility had more in-person votes per capita than states with higher election flexibility. A one-unit increase in the election flexibility score reduced long in-person visits by 155 per 100,000 votes cast.[2] The estimate is statistically significant at a 90-percent confidence level and suggests that such processes as remote and early voting lower polling station congestion and reduce the number of lengthy, high-risk visits.

We also use this model and estimation technique to test the effect of election flexibility on all polling station visits—not just long ones. Election flexibility is again negatively correlated with in-person voting: Our model predicts that a one-unit increase in election flexibility score lowered the incidence of in-person voting by 267 per 100,000 votes, which is also statisti-

---

[2]   The coefficient, 0.09, is the effect of a one-unit increase in the election flexibility score on the standard deviation of the per capita long-visits variable. The standard deviation of the long-visits variable is 0.01, or 1 percent of the county's population. Thus, the average marginal effect estimate is 1% × 0.09 = 0.09%.

cally significant. Flexible election processes appear to be strongly correlated with lower congestion at polling stations in 2020.

Estimating the Effect of In-Person Voting on COVID-19 Transmission

We now address our second question about in-person voting: To what extent did in-person voting accelerate transmission of COVID-19? To answer this question, we compare the spread of COVID-19 in counties with higher rates of per capita in-person voting on Election Day with the spread of COVID-19 in counties with lower in-person voting rates. We track COVID-19 spread using the Johns Hopkins Center for Systems Science and Engineering (CSSE) data, which lists new COVID-19 cases for each U.S. county.

Figure 4.4 plots the seven-day moving average of states' cases over time.[3] Each panel in Figure 4.4 corresponds to one of the four election flexibility categories: very low (top left), low (top right), medium (bottom left), and high (bottom right). Not all states are included in this analysis because not all states report their polling locations to CPI, while others, such as New Jersey, did not hold in-person elections at all so there was simply no polling station data to share. States that qualify for the analysis have their initials listed in bold and their new COVID-19 cases plotted in their respective panel.

The data used in the following analysis are at the county-week level and contains the total number of new COVID-19 cases per capita and the total number of long Election-Day visits per capita for each county.[4] The data cover 2,154 counties (of 2,220 possible counties) in 34 states across 19 weeks (i.e., nine weeks before the election, election week, and nine weeks after the election).[5]

---

[3]   Although state averages are plotted, the data are built from the same county-level data used in the analysis that follows.

[4]   County-level population data come from the 2019 American Community Survey from the Integrated Public Use Microdata Series.

[5]   For reference, there are 3,006 counties in the United States.

FIGURE 4.4

New COVID-19 Cases per Capita by Election Flexibility Category

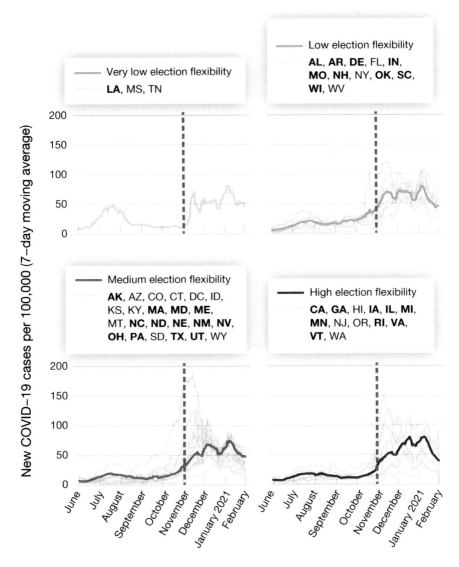

SOURCE: Features CSSE data.
NOTE: States that qualify for the analysis have their initials listed in bold and their new COVID-19 cases plotted in their respective panel.

In this setting, the treatment date is the presidential election, which took place in all counties on November 3, 2020, and the treatment is the in-person votes per capita, which, of course, varied by county.[6] We suspected that counties with more in-person per capita voting would have higher rates of per capita COVID-19 transmission in the following nine weeks. Two models were employed to test this hypothesis: difference-in-differences and event study. Both models included county and week dummy variables: the former controlled for both observed and unobserved time-invariant county-specific characteristics that might affect their rate of COVID-19 infection (e.g., higher population density, income, age, racial composition),[7] while the latter controlled for systematic differences, both observed and unobserved, between the time units, which, in this case, was weeks. These two components (i.e., county and week dummy variables) were the elements that we relied on to identify the causal effect of in-person voting: The identification strategy did not vary between models. (We refer the reader to the box in Chapter 2 that explains the intuition behind difference-in-differences, fixed effects, and event study designs.)

We use two models, difference-in-differences and event study, because each one tells us something different about the relationship between in-person voting and COVID-19 spread. Difference-in-differences estimates the **average** effect of per capita in-person voting across the entire following nine weeks, while the event study model allows us to observe the effect over time. Difference-in-differences produces a single estimated effect, while event study designs produce an estimated effect for each period, which, in our case, is each week before and after the election. The week of the election serves as a baseline and effects are estimated relative to it.

---

[6] A single common treatment period (e.g., November 3) does not introduce bias that arises in difference-in-differences or TWFE models with *staggered* treatment, a relatively recent development in the econometrics literature. See Goodman-Bacon, 2021 for an explanation of this bias and ways to address it.

[7] We point out that these are not controls included in the model, but they are also the sort of variables that need not be included because the fixed effect already controls for their influence.

Relationship of In-Person Voting and Number of New COVID-19 Cases

Figure 4.5 plots the 18 event study coefficients over the 19 weeks in our analysis and the bounds for statistical significance. There are nine pre-election weeks used in the analysis but only eight coefficients because the week preceding the election is omitted from the model, following standard event study regression design. The ten remaining coefficients cover the week of the election and the nine weeks that follow. The red dashed line indicates the average effect estimate across the entire period using the difference-in-differences model.

The event study coefficients (black squares) give the estimated effect of in-person voting on the number of new COVID-19 cases. The average effect estimate, from the model, is 0.026, meaning that for each additional long visit to polling station on Election Day, there were 0.026 new COVID-19

FIGURE 4.5

In-Person Voting's Effect on COVID-19 Spread

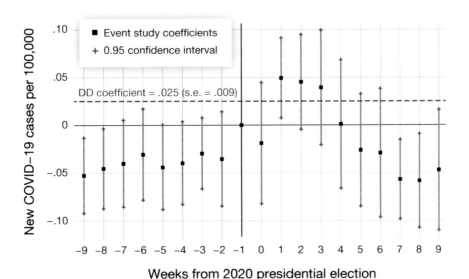

SOURCE: Features CSSE data.

cases in the nine weeks following the election. The event study coefficients, plotted as black squares, are the estimated effects for each week. Their *whiskers*, the gray lines that extend above and below them, show their 95-percent confidence interval. When they intersect with 0 on the y-axis, the effects are statistically insignificant. The eight pre-election coefficients should be statistically indistinguishable from 0 because the election should not have affected the spread of COVID-19 in the past. If we detect sizable estimated effects before the election, it raises concerns about the validity of the empirical design. In our case, the estimated pre-election coefficients are less than 0 in three of the eight pre-treatment coefficients. We observe strong, positive effects that peak in the first week after the election, at about 0.05 new cases per additional visit, return to 0 by the fourth week, and become negative for the remainder of the post-treatment period.

Chapter Summary

This chapter estimated the effects of flexible election processes and policies on public health in a two-part analysis.

The first analysis tested whether flexible voting laws lowered the incidence of in-person voting. This analysis found that states with greater flexibility saw lower rates of long visits (i.e., those lasting longer than 20 minutes) and of all visits regardless of duration. Our statistical model found that a one-unit increase in a state's election flexibility score led to 155 fewer long visits per 100,000 votes cast.

The second analysis showed that long visits incurred significant costs to public health. We empirically tested this hypothesis by comparing the spread of COVID-19 in counties with different levels of in-person voting per capita. We estimate that each additional visit led to 0.026 additional COVID-19 cases in the nine weeks after the election. Had all Americans voted remotely, the model predicts there would have been roughly 500,000 fewer new cases of COVID-19 in the ten weeks following the election.

The precision of such calculations is fraught. The calculations rely on our estimates, which in turn depend on assumptions that are, in some cases, impossible to test and on imperfect data. Despite these caveats, the robust trends we examine between election flexibility, in-person voting, and the spread of COVID-19 suggest that there is a significant public health cost imposed by inflexible voting processes.

CHAPTER 5

Concluding Thoughts

In this report, we tested whether flexible state election processes improved turnout or mitigated the spread of COVID-19 after the 2020 election. The analysis shows that there are sizable benefits to flexible election processes, particularly when faced with a pandemic that imposes risks to in-person voting at crowded polls. Previous research exploring the effects of voting processes (e.g., no-excuse absentee ballots) demonstrated that their use produced only mild improvements in voter turnout; these results are consistent with the theory that the costs of voting in person are small relative to voting's benefits. Although our report similarly finds only mild effects on total turnout, we show that prior studies do not fully capture the effects of flexible voting processes, which were also manifest in the increased use of absentee ballots, which, in turn, reduced the spread of COVID-19 by lowering congestion at polling stations in the 2020 election.

This report is not a full cost-benefit analysis of election processes. We do not closely examine the financial costs that many laws and processes entail, or whether absentee ballots lead to greater incidence of voter fraud—though extant research shows voter fraud to be an exceptionally rare phenomenon, whether the ballot is cast in person or mailed in (Bump, 2016; Hood and Gillespie, 2012; Wu et al., 2020).

With that caveat aside, the report does identify and, to the extent possible, quantify three effects of flexible voting laws: (1) large increases in voter turnout, (2) reductions in in-person voting on Election Day, and (3) slower spread of COVID-19 in the weeks after the election.

At the same time, our analysis suggests that the efficacy of flexible election policies depends on the public's willingness to utilize them. Demographic groups that expressed skepticism around the security and safety of absentee ballots were far less responsive to changes in their state's voting law flexibility.

State legislatures should weigh these benefits as they assess the many proposals to change voting. Policymakers, pundits, and political leaders might be able to improve their efficacy through positive public messaging and, for policymakers, by increasing the transparency and security of the absentee ballot and early voting processes—though the precise extent to which these strategies might increase the use of flexible election processes falls outside the scope of this report.

Technical Details

In this appendix, we detail the technical aspects of our statistical analysis throughout the report. For each analysis, we write out its empirical model and explain the technique used to estimate the model parameters. This appendix also includes tables of all the parameters' estimates and additional regression statistics. The analyses are presented in the same order as they appear in the report.

The Effects of State Election Processes on Voters' Behavior—Technical Appendix (Chapter 3)

In Chapter 3, we explore the effect of election flexibility on voting turnout and voting method. The first analysis uses data from MEDSL, which lists U.S. counties, their total votes cast, and votes cast for the Republican and Democratic candidates for the 2012, 2016, and 2020 elections. The analysis tests whether election flexibility scores affect voter turnout in the 2020 general election. To test this hypothesis, we construct an empirical model, which includes county (ϕ_c) and election fixed effects (γ_t):

$$y_{ct} = \beta_0 f_{st} + \gamma_t + \phi_c + \epsilon_{ct}.$$

The dependent variable (y_{ct}) changes throughout the analysis. In the first column of Table A.1, the dependent variable (or outcome) is total votes cast in county (c), in election (t). To measure the responsiveness of Democrats and Republicans individually, the dependent variable becomes simply votes for the Democratic presidential candidate and Republican candidates in columns two and three, respectively. The numerator of this variable comes from MEDSL data, while the denominator (i.e., the county's population) comes from the census' five-year ACS via NHGIS's data portal (Manson et al., 2021). The model includes a constant term (α) and both county (ϕ_c) and election (γ_t) fixed effects. The coefficient of interest is β_0, which estimates the effect of a change in a state's election flexibility score; f_{st} takes the value of each county's election flexibility score, which varies by state (s), in the 2020 election year, and is 0 in earlier elections. Table A.1 presents the results of those three regressions using the model described above.

In Chapter 3 we estimate the decrease of votes for Joe Biden in the 2020 election had states lowered their election flexibility score by one. This box illustrates the calculation. The model, explained above, yields an estimate of an increase of 1.2 percentage points of Democrats' vote share for a one-unit increase in the election flexibility score. There were 31,983,911 votes for Biden in states with high election flexibility, 27,786,079 in medium election flexibility states and 18,372,649 in low flexibility states. To calculate the reduction in votes for Joe Biden, we sum these numbers and multiply by 0.012 (1.2%) to arrive at a figure of 937,712 fewer votes.

TABLE A.1
Election Flexibility and Voter Turnout

Coefficient Estimate	All Votes	Democratic Votes	Republican Votes
Election flexibility	0.009*	0.012***	−0.003
	(0.005)	(0.003)	(0.002)
Number of observations	9,330	9,330	9,330
R-squared	0.949	0.947	0.963

NOTE: This table presents estimates of election flexibility on voter turnout. It uses a panel data of 3,110 U.S. counties' votes in the 2012, 2016, and 2020 elections. The parameters are estimated using an ordinary least squares regression (from the Stata command "reghdfe") with county and election fixed effects. In columns two and three, we use only the number of votes for the Democratic and Republican candidates, respectively. The coefficient of interest is election flexibility, which gives the effect of a one-unit increase in the election flexibility score on voter turnout. Significance levels are indicated: * 10%, ** 5%, and *** 1%.

Interpreting the coefficients is straightforward. Ordinary least squares regression coefficients tell the predicted change in the dependent variable for a one-unit change in the independent variable. In this case, the coefficients tell us how an increase in a state's election flexibility score predicts changes in voter turnout: an increase in the score corresponds to a 0.9 percentage point increase in the percentage of the county's residence casting a ballot and a 1.2 percentage point increase in votes for the Democratic party's candidate.

This model treats the election flexibility score as a continuous predictor variable. However, the election flexibility index is not continuous but an ordered categorical variable. It takes one of four discrete values: very low (0), low (1), medium (2), and high (3). Researchers often face the question of whether to treat a variable as continuous or as ordered categorical in their empirical models. The decision rests on whether the categorical variable has many discrete values, in which case empiricists often treat it as a continuous variable. Three values are often considered the bare minimum for treating a categorical variable as continuous, and the election flexibility includes only four ordered values. For this reason, in the main report, we treated the measure as continuous in the empirical models. Here, we take the alternative approach and include each flexibility score as its own predictor in the model. The single continuous variable is replaced by three dummy (i.e., binary or dichotomous) variables that equal 1 when the state's election flexibility score is equal to the score that the dummy captures in the treatment year (i.e., 2020). The dummies are 0 in the pre-treatment years. The very low flexibility score is the omitted category and states with low, medium, and high flexibility are compared with the very low group. The specification is as follows:

$$y_{ct} = \alpha_0 + \sum_{i=1}^{3} \beta_i f i_{st} + \gamma_t + \phi_c + \epsilon_{ct}.$$

The dependent variable and fixed effects are identical to the previous model specification—the only difference is that we have added the three dummy variables discussed above: $f1_{st}, f2_{st}, f3_{st}$, for the low, medium, and high flexibility states, respectively. Table A.2 contains the results for this regression and reveals some nonlinearity in the effects. Although the beneficial effects of flexible election processes on turnout monotonically increase,

TABLE A.2

Election Flexibility and Voter Turnout (Nonlinear)

Coefficient Estimate	All Votes	Democratic Votes	Republican Votes
Low election flexibility	0.015	0.012	0.008
	(0.020)	(0.009)	(0.012)
Medium election flexibility	0.029	0.029***	0.004
	(0.020)	(0.010)	(0.012)
High election flexibility	0.032	0.037***	−0.000
	(0.019)	(0.010)	(0.011)
Number of observations	9,330	9,330	9,330
R-squared	0.949	0.947	0.963

NOTE: This table presents estimates of election flexibility on voter turnout. It uses a panel data of 3,110 U.S. counties' votes in the 2012, 2016, and 2020 elections. The parameters are estimated using an ordinary least squares regression (from the Stata command reghdfe) with county and election fixed effects. In columns two and three, we use only the number of votes for the Democratic and Republican candidates, respectively. The coefficients of interest are the election flexibility dummies for the low, medium, and high election flexibility states. These coefficients tell the effect of counties switching to the respective election flexibility category from the very low category, which is the omitted group. Significance levels are indicated: * 10%, ** 5%, and *** 1%.

there are substantial differences between very low flexibility states (i.e., the omitted category) and all other states, another large gap between low and medium/high states (approximately a 1.5 percentage point jump) but relatively little difference between the impacts felt by medium-high states, which had turnout around 3 percentage points higher than the very low flexibility states. The results suggest that not all election flexibility dimensions (i.e., voter registration, early voting, and remote voting) have identical impacts on voters' behaviors. However, we do not investigate the effects of individual voting laws on turnout in this paper. Again, we observe much stronger effects among Democratic voters than among Republican voters.

In this section, we test the effect of election processes on voting method using Aristotle's consumer data file. These data, unlike MEDSL's election data, are a cross section. In other words, we observe the behavior of voters only in the 2020 election and not the ones preceding it. To estimate the effect of election processes on voting method, we construct another empirical model that includes several variables that we suspect also influence voters' decisions about which method to use when casting their ballot (e.g., political affiliation, sex, age, net worth). These data for the control variables also come from Aristotle's consumer data file and vary at the individual level. All the variables are categorical. For example, individuals' net worth falls into bins, ranging from < $0 to > $499,999. Table A.3 lists the categories in their entirety.

The empirical model we use to estimate the effect of flexible election processes on voter's voting method is as follows:

$$y_i = \alpha + \beta_1 f_s + X'_i \pi + \epsilon_i.$$

The coefficient of interest is β_1 and captures the estimated effect of state election processes on voting method. It includes a vector of controls (X'_i) that are listed above. The outcome, y_i, is the method that voters use to cast their ballot and it is categorical. Voters do one of four things in the 2020 election: (1) vote remotely, (2) vote early, (3) vote on Election Day, or (4) abstain. For a categorical dependent variable, we use a multinomial logit model designed for categorical outcomes (i.e., the command "*mlogit*" in Stata). The results are listed in Table A.3. The first panel presents estimates of a simple bivariate model, which does not include any controls. Controls are added in the second panel, where their coefficients and standard errors, which are clustered at the state level, are also listed. We use the identical model specification to estimate the effects for each race or ethnicity. We use stratified samples that include only the voters identified as each race or ethnicity and again use multinomial logit models to estimate effects by race/ethnicity. The results are listed in Table A.4.

State Election Policy and COVID-19 Spread— Technical Appendix (Chapter 4)

Chapter 4 explores the effects of (1) election flexibility scores on the incidence of long visits to polling stations (i.e., those lasting longer than 20 minutes) and (2) how long visits affect the spread of COVID-19 in the election's wake.

TABLE A.3

Effect of Election Processes on Voting Method

Voting Method	Absentee	Election Day	Early
Model 1: Bivariate			
Election flexibility	0.874***	−0.158	−0.311
	(0.260)	(0.160)	(0.286)
Number of observations			167,513,505
Pseudo R-*squared*			0.0484
Model 2: Controls for ethnicity, party affiliation, gender, age, and net worth			
Election flexibility	0.902**	−0.135	−0.306
	(0.277)	(0.149)	(0.296)
Asian	omitted	omitted	omitted
Black	0.151	0.449**	0.706
	(0.184)	(0.137)	(0.414)
Hispanic	0.0550	−0.0247	0.639**
	(0.187)	(0.149)	(0.201)
Native	0.143	0.352	1.197**
	(0.301)	(0.265)	(0.458)
Pacific islander	−0.0477	−0.0261	0.103
	(0.162)	(0.136)	(0.218)
Unknown race/ethnicity	0.436**	0.793***	0.205
	(0.161)	(0.101)	(0.190)
White	0.451*	0.701***	0.595
	(0.180)	(0.120)	(0.310)
Democrat	omitted	omitted	omitted
Independent	−0.388*	−0.318	−0.471
	(0.158)	(0.229)	(0.457)
Nonpartisan	−0.234	−0.327	−0.155
	(0.213)	(0.229)	(0.377)
Republican	−0.214*	0.340***	0.363**
	(0.0946)	(0.0720)	(0.116)
Unknown	−1.090***	−0.196	−0.666
	(0.262)	(0.161)	(0.450)

Table A.3—Continued

Voting Method	Absentee	Election Day	Early
Female	omitted	omitted	omitted
Male	−0.138***	−0.0313**	−0.0959***
	(0.0188)	(0.0115)	(0.0228)
Unknown sex	−0.242***	−0.252***	−0.183*
	(0.0345)	(0.0320)	(0.0836)
Age	0.0188***	0.00580**	0.00889**
	(0.00230)	(0.00207)	(0.00287)
Unknown net worth	omitted	omitted	omitted
Net worth: < $1	−0.782***	−0.362***	−0.655***
	(0.0696)	(0.0522)	(0.121)
$1–$4,999	−0.674***	0.131**	−0.301
	(0.108)	(0.0500)	(0.155)
$5,000–$9,999	−0.467***	0.142***	−0.168
	(0.0860)	(0.0405)	(0.111)
$10,000–$24,999	−0.468***	0.195***	−0.124
	(0.0942)	(0.0450)	(0.118)
$25,000–$49,999	−0.331***	0.213***	−0.0550
	(0.0825)	(0.0398)	(0.0963)
$50,000–$99,999	−0.200**	0.222***	−0.0163
	(0.0742)	(0.0417)	(0.0831)
$100,000–$249,999	0.0896	0.287***	0.0726
	(0.0686)	(0.0488)	(0.0818)
$250,000–$499,999	0.332***	0.302***	0.0987
	(0.0798)	(0.0651)	(0.111)
> $499,999	0.590***	0.328**	0.111
	(0.111)	(0.106)	(0.187)
Number of observations			165,927,899
Pseudo R-*squared*			0.0892

NOTE: This table presents the coefficient estimates from a categorical logit regression. The omitted outcome (i.e., the base outcome) is abstention and the alternative outcomes are absentee, early, and Election-Day voting. The coefficient of interest is the state's election flexibility score. Significance levels are indicated: * 10%, ** 5%, and *** 1%.

TABLE A.4

Effect of Election Processes on Voting Method by Race or Ethnicity

Coefficient Estimate	Panel A: Asian Voters			Panel B: Black Voters		
	Absentee	Election Day	Early	Absentee	Election Day	Early
Election flexibility	0.988*	−0.283	−0.578	0.905**	−0.252	−0.0536
	(0.391)	(0.201)	(0.377)	(0.347)	(0.179)	(0.332)
Democrat	–	–	–	–	–	–
Independent	−0.219	−0.205	−0.513	−0.364	−0.349*	−1.155***
	(0.205)	(0.222)	(0.593)	(0.214)	(0.170)	(0.350)
Nonpartisan	−0.177	−0.248	−0.327	−0.235	−0.735***	−0.00682
	(0.192)	(0.220)	(0.533)	(0.188)	(0.169)	(0.211)
Republican	−0.332*	0.252	0.569*	−0.251	0.271**	−0.116
	(0.148)	(0.138)	(0.242)	(0.156)	(0.0853)	(0.210)
Unknown	−1.155***	−0.0166	0.459	−0.977***	−0.219	−1.401
	(0.288)	(0.213)	(0.458)	(0.196)	(0.131)	(0.743)
Female	–	–	–	–	–	–
Male	−0.0374	0.0137	−0.0381	−0.360***	−0.282***	−0.360***
	(0.0222)	(0.0148)	(0.0228)	(0.0335)	(0.0154)	(0.0355)
Unknown sex	−0.0305	0.0123	0.0814	−0.291***	−0.254***	−0.411***
	(0.114)	(0.0822)	(0.0959)	(0.0408)	(0.0321)	(0.107)
Age	0.00289	−0.00154	−0.00185	0.0253***	0.0105***	0.0124**
	(0.00483)	(0.00366)	(0.00359)	(0.00325)	(0.00310)	(0.00466)
Unknown net worth	–	–	–	–	–	–
Net worth: <$1	−0.714***	−0.397***	−0.759***	−0.653***	−0.288***	−0.387*
	(0.0698)	(0.0591)	(0.132)	(0.0738)	(0.0706)	(0.178)

Table A.4—Continued

Coefficient Estimate	Panel A: Asian Voters			Panel B: Black Voters		
	Absentee	Election Day	Early	Absentee	Election Day	Early
$1–$4,999	−0.439***	0.130	−0.337	−0.0945	0.290***	0.257
	(0.116)	(0.0852)	(0.252)	(0.117)	(0.0601)	(0.209)
$5,000–$9,999	−0.404***	−0.00323	−0.282	0.0171	0.234***	0.366*
	(0.0864)	(0.0615)	(0.193)	(0.0852)	(0.0577)	(0.158)
$10,000–$24,999	−0.407***	0.0571	−0.218	0.0361	0.269***	0.390*
	(0.0907)	(0.0575)	(0.176)	(0.0914)	(0.0569)	(0.169)
$25,000–$49,999	−0.384***	0.00913	−0.170	0.152*	0.266***	0.515***
	(0.0676)	(0.0504)	(0.0995)	(0.0731)	(0.0607)	(0.145)
$50,000–$99,999	−0.298***	0.00346	−0.116	0.195**	0.215***	0.478***
	(0.0549)	(0.0518)	(0.0704)	(0.0668)	(0.0608)	(0.139)
$100,000–$249,999	−0.168**	−0.0163	−0.118	0.536***	0.268***	0.648***
	(0.0587)	(0.0653)	(0.0663)	(0.0685)	(0.0716)	(0.142)
$250,000–$499,999	0.0307	0.0411	−0.0320	0.737***	0.266***	0.541*
	(0.0626)	(0.0685)	(0.0875)	(0.127)	(0.0782)	(0.217)
>$499,999	0.222*	0.0876	−0.230	0.913***	0.283**	0.412
	(0.106)	(0.108)	(0.174)	(0.168)	(0.105)	(0.285)
Number of observations	4,842,934			12,357,847		
Pseudo R–squared	0.0959			0.0859		

Table A.4—Continued

Coefficient Estimate	Panel C: Hispanic Voters			Panel D: White Voters		
	Absentee	Election day	Early	Absentee	Election day	Early
Election flexibility	0.823*	−0.115	−0.478	0.913***	−0.119	−0.317
	(0.358)	(0.219)	(0.360)	(0.265)	(0.145)	(0.302)
Democrat	–	–	–	–	–	–
Independent	−0.266	−0.249	−0.460	−0.418**	−0.328	−0.447
	(0.240)	(0.223)	(0.402)	(0.161)	(0.242)	(0.484)
Nonpartisan	−0.0834	−0.308	−0.659	−0.253	−0.302	−0.0433
	(0.260)	(0.202)	(0.418)	(0.243)	(0.248)	(0.392)
Republican	0.0772	0.362***	0.501**	−0.231*	0.345***	0.389***
	(0.100)	(0.105)	(0.176)	(0.104)	(0.0804)	(0.113)
Unknown	−1.619***	−0.279	−0.257	−1.041***	−0.177	−0.759
	(0.360)	(0.179)	(0.236)	(0.276)	(0.185)	(0.458)
Female	–	–	–	–	–	–
Male	−0.225***	−0.151***	−0.153***	−0.104***	0.00825	−0.0594**
	(0.0181)	(0.0202)	(0.0216)	(0.0182)	(0.0123)	(0.0227)
Unknown sex	−0.193***	−0.147***	−0.245***	−0.274***	−0.288***	−0.176
	(0.0301)	(0.0219)	(0.0400)	(0.0358)	(0.0396)	(0.0918)
Age	0.0150***	0.00216	0.00535*	0.0196***	0.00605**	0.00939**
	(0.00203)	(0.00261)	(0.00268)	(0.00240)	(0.00204)	(0.00292)
Unknown net worth	–	–	–	–	–	–
Net worth: <$1	−0.553***	−0.255***	−0.683***	−0.795***	−0.387***	−0.627***
	(0.107)	(0.0552)	(0.141)	(0.0762)	(0.0563)	(0.135)
$1–$4,999	−0.656***	−0.146	0.0594	−0.768***	0.110*	−0.445*
	(0.194)	(0.142)	(0.121)	(0.121)	(0.0526)	(0.178)

Table A.4—Continued

Coefficient Estimate	Panel C: Hispanic Voters			Panel D: White Voters		
	Absentee	Election day	Early	Absentee	Election day	Early
$5,000–$9,999	−0.441**	−0.0822	0.0620	−0.509***	0.151***	−0.261*
	(0.152)	(0.107)	(0.0779)	(0.0926)	(0.0394)	(0.128)
$10,000–$24,999	−0.485**	−0.100	0.106	−0.504***	0.215***	−0.211
	(0.158)	(0.109)	(0.0828)	(0.101)	(0.0426)	(0.137)
$25,000–$49,999	−0.263**	0.0263	0.147**	−0.368***	0.225***	−0.132
	(0.101)	(0.0739)	(0.0482)	(0.0915)	(0.0398)	(0.110)
$50,000–$99,999	−0.119	0.0719	0.155**	−0.229**	0.236***	−0.0735
	(0.0761)	(0.0713)	(0.0508)	(0.0828)	(0.0428)	(0.0921)
$100,000–$249,999	0.235***	0.229***	0.139	0.0607	0.298***	0.0383
	(0.0704)	(0.0638)	(0.0979)	(0.0779)	(0.0544)	(0.0847)
$250,000–$499,999	0.501***	0.326**	0.0301	0.310***	0.309***	0.0909
	(0.137)	(0.101)	(0.190)	(0.0873)	(0.0723)	(0.107)
>$499,999	0.762***	0.507***	−0.0533	0.593***	0.341**	0.133
	(0.164)	(0.145)	(0.270)	(0.120)	(0.112)	(0.185)
Number of observations		15,955,781			123,803,628	
Pseudo R-*squared*		0.0832			0.0851	

NOTE: This table presents the coefficient estimates from a categorical logit regression where the outcome is voters' choice of voting method. There are four possible outcomes: absentee, early voting, Election-Day voting, and abstention. The omitted outcomes (i.e., the base outcome) is abstention. The coefficient of interest is the state's election flexibility score. "Democrat," "Female," and "Unknown net worth" are the omitted categories for political party, sex, and net worth, which is indicated by dashes in those rows. Each panel presents estimates for one of the four racial or ethnic groups for whom we estimate effects (i.e., Asian, Black, Hispanic, and White voters). Significance levels are indicated: * 10%, ** 5%, and *** 1%.

To estimate the first effect, we use a cross section of data stitched together from: (1) RAND's election flexibility index, (2) SafeGraph's cell phone location data and CPI's 2020 polling location data to develop estimates of long visits per capita, (3) population, demographic, and county area data from the ACS, and (4) the MEDSL's election data, which include the number of votes for Donald Trump and Joe Biden, the Republican and Democratic candidates respectively. The data's sources and cleaning are described in greater detail in Chapter 4. We use the following model to estimate the effect. As we mention in the main body of the text, the identification of the causal effect is difficult to obtain in this setting. The treatment, flexible election processes, is not assigned randomly and, although we attempt to control for confounding variables (i.e., its share of Black voters, population density, total number of polls, and Republican vote share per capita), this approach does not control for all potential confounders. For this reason, the findings should be treated as conditional correlations rather than causal effects.

$$y_i = \alpha + \beta_2 f_s + X_i' \tau + \epsilon_i.$$

In this model, y_i is the number of long visits to polling stations in each U.S. county per 100,000 votes cast, although α again serves as an intercept. In a second specification, the dependent variable is the total number of visits per 100,000 votes cast. The coefficient of interest in this model is β_2 which estimates the average effect of an increase in a state's election flexibility score. The preceding paragraph lists the controls that are included in the vector, X_i'. Finally, ϵ_i is the model's error term. Table A.5 contains the raw coefficients from the model.

In this specification, we again treat the election flexibility index as a continuous variable. As we did in our technical appendix material for Chapter 3 above, we re-create the model replacing the single, continuous flexibility measure with a collection of dummy variables indicating whether a county belongs in the low, medium, or high election flexibility categories. Model 1 still includes all controls and Model 2 includes only the three dummy variables. We test the effects on both dependent variables: long and all polling station visits. The estimates can be found in Table A.6, where we observe some nonlinearity in the effects, driven by the very low flexibility group (i.e., Louisiana), whose polls were much less congested than polls in counties with low flexibility. Moderate and high flexibility states still had the least

TABLE A.5

Election Flexibility and In–Person Voting

Coefficient Estimate	Long Visits per 100,000 Votes		All Visits per 100,000 Votes	
Independent Variables	Model 1	Model 2	Model 1	Model 2
Election flexibility	−154.6**	−144.2**	−267.4**	−261.0*
	(57.78)	(60.99)	(129.6)	(138.3)
Income per capita	0.102		0.0534	
	(0.0699)		(0.0596)	
Black population share	−402.1		−557.2	
	(241.2)		(485.9)	
Population density	−13,628.6		−45,887.0	
	(28,934.2)		(68,880.3)	
Number of polls	0.921***		0.943***	
	(0.298)		(0.291)	
Republican votes per capita	419.1		1,740.5**	
	(298.8)		(725.1)	
Number of observations	2,135	2,135	2,135	2,135
R-squared	0.07	0.03	0.06	0.03

NOTE: Model 1 includes all controls, while Model 2 is a simple bivariate regression. There are two outcome variables: long visits to polling stations on Election Day per capita and all visits per capita. Significance levels are indicated: * 10%, ** 5%, and *** 1%.

congested polls, but the benefits of moderate flexibility (relative to very low) are not statistically significant in any model specification.

In the second section of Chapter 4, we test the effect of long visits to polling stations on Election Day per 100,000 people on the number of new COVID-19 cases per 100,000 people. Unlike the first analysis, where we have only a cross section to identify the effect of the treatment (i.e., elec-

TABLE A.6

Election Flexibility and In–Person Voting (Nonlinear)

	Run 1	Run 2	Run 3
Coefficient estimate	All votes	Democratic votes	Republican votes
Low election flexibility	0.015	0.012	0.008
	(0.020)	(0.009)	(0.012)
Medium election flexibility	0.029	0.029***	0.004
	(0.020)	(0.010)	(0.012)
High election flexibility	0.032	0.037***	−0.000
	(0.019)	(0.010)	(0.011)
Number of observations	9,330	9,330	9,330
R-squared	0.949	0.947	0.963

NOTE: Model 1 includes all controls, while Model 2 is a simple bivariate regression. There are two outcome variables: long visits to polling stations on Election Day per capita and all visits per capita. Here, we treated election flexibility as a set of dummy variables. The very low election flexibility counties are the omitted group, to which all other categories (i.e., low, medium, and high) are compared. Significance levels are indicated: * 10%, ** 5%, and *** 1%.

tion flexibility scores), here, we use a panel of data that tracks the new COVID-19 cases in each U.S. county for each week. The data are at the U.S. county week level and include information on each county's long visits per 100,000 people. The model does not include any control variables. Instead, it identifies the effect of visits by using difference-in-differences and event study identification strategies. The difference-in-differences model has the following specification:

$$y_{ct} = \beta_3 l_c + \gamma_t + \phi_c + \epsilon_{ct}.$$

The event study specification adds terms for each pretreatment and post-treatment period except for the week directly preceding the election. Its specification is as follows:

$$y_{ct} = \sum_{j=2}^{J} \beta_j (Lag\, j)_{ct} + \sum_{k=1}^{K} \beta_k (Lead\, k)_{ct} + \gamma_t + \phi_c + \epsilon_{ct}.$$

We model the behavior of new COVID-19 cases, y, in county c in week t. J indexes the eight pre-treatment dummies and K the 10 post-treatment week dummies. These terms take the value of the counties' election flexibility scores in the week they index, allowing us to track the evolution of in-person voting's effect on new COVID-19 cases. y_t and ϕ_c are the time and county fixed effects. α is the intercept term and ϵ_{ct} the idiosyncratic error term.

The results from the difference-in-differences and event study regressions can be found in Tables A.7 and A.8 respectively.

In Chapter 4 we estimate the total number of COVID-19 cases that might have been avoided had the election been held remotely. The calculation is explained here: 155 million people voted in the election. Around 27 percent (approximately 41.85 million people) voted in person on Election Day. Our SafeGraph data show that approximately 47 percent of all polling station visits were long, meaning that there were 19.8 million long visits on Election Day. We estimate that 2.6 percent of visits led to a new COVID-19 case, meaning that, had the election been held remotely, the United States might have been able to avoid approximately 500,000 new cases of COVID-19 in the ten weeks following the election.

TABLE A.7

In–Person Voting and COVID–19 (Difference–in–Differences)

Coefficient Estimate	New COVID–19 Cases per 100,000
Long waits per 100,000	0.026
	(0.009)
County FE	Yes
Week FE	Yes
Number of observations	40,926
R-*squared*	0.269

NOTE: FE = fixed effects.

TABLE A.8

In–Person Voting and COVID–19 (Event Study)

Week to Election	Effect	Week to Election	Effect
−9	−0.053***	1	0.049**
	(0.020)		(0.021)
−8	−0.046**	2	0.045*
	(0.021)		(0.025)
−7	−0.040*	3	0.039
	(0.023)		(0.031)
−6	−0.031	4	0.001
	(0.024)		(0.034)
−5	−0.044**	5	−0.026
	(0.022)		(0.030)
−4	−0.040*	6	−0.028
	(0.022)		(0.034)
−3	−0.030	7	−0.056***
	(0.019)		(0 .021)
−2	−0.036	8	−0.058**
	(0.025)		(0.025)
0	−0.018	9	−0.046
	(0.032)		(0.032)
County FE		Yes	
Week FE		Yes	
Number of observations		40,926	
R-*squared*		0.267	

NOTE: Significance levels are indicated: * 10%, ** 5%, and *** 1%.

Abbreviations

ACS	American Community Survey
AVR	automatic voter registration
COVID-19	coronavirus disease 2019
CPI	Center for Public Integrity
CSSE	Center for Systems Science and Engineering
FE	fixed effects
MEDSL	MIT Election Data and Science Lab
NCF	National Consumer File
NHGIS	National Historical Geographic Information System
POIs	places of interest
TWFE	two-way fixed effects

References

Ballotpedia, "Election Policy: Enlightening Voters on Policy Matters," webpage, undated. As of January 1, 2023:
https://ballotpedia.org/Election_Policy

Bump, Philip, "There Have Been Just Four Documented Cases of Voter Fraud in the 2016 Election," *Washington Post*, December 1, 2016.

Burden, Barry C., David T. Canon, Kenneth R. Mayer, and Donald P. Moynihan, "Election Laws, Mobilization, and Turnout: The Unanticipated Consequences of Election Reform," *American Journal of Political Science*, Vol. 58, No. 1, 2014.

Cantoni, Enrico, and Vincent Pons, "Strict ID Laws Don't Stop Voters: Evidence from a U.S. Nationwide Panel, 2008–2018," *Quarterly Journal of Economics*, Vol. 136, No. 4, 2021.

Centers for Disease Control and Prevention, "Quarantine and Isolation," webpage, January 27, 2022. As of March 22, 2022:
https://www.cdc.gov/coronavirus/2019-ncov/your-health/quarantine-isolation.html

Chen, M. Keith, Kareem Haggag, Devin G. Pope, and Ryne Rohla, "Racial Disparities in Voting Wait Times: Evidence from Smartphone Data," *Review of Economics and Statistics*, Vol. 104, No. 6, 2020.

Chou, Sophie, and Tyler Dukes, "In North Carolina, Black Voters' Mail-In Ballots Much More Likely to Be Rejected Than Those from Any Other Race," ProPublica, September 23, 2020.

Clinton, Joshua D., Nick Eubank, Adriane Fresh, and Michael E. Shepherd, "Polling Place Changes and Political Participation: Evidence from North Carolina Presidential Elections, 2008–2016," *Political Science Research and Methods*, Vol. 9, No. 4, 2020.

Cohut, Maria, "US Election 2020: Many People Concerned About COVID-19 Risk," *Medical News Today*, October 2, 2020.

Cotti, Chad, Bryan Engelhardt, Joshua Foster, Erik Nesson, and Paul Niekamp, "The Relationship Between In-Person Voting and COVID-19: Evidence from the Wisconsin Primary," *Contemporary Economic Policy*, Vol. 39, No. 4, January 14, 2021.

DeSilver, Drew, "Turnout Soared in 2020 as Nearly Two-Thirds of Eligible U.S. Voters Cast Ballots for President," Pew Research Center, January 28, 2021.

Feltham, Eric M., Laura Forastiere, Marcus Alexander, and Nicholas A. Christakis, "No Increase in COVID-19 Mortality After the 2020 Primary Elections in the USA," *arXiv*, October 8, 2020.

Goodman-Bacon, Andrew, "Difference-in-Differences with Variation in Treatment Timing," *Journal of Econometrics*, Vol. 225, No. 2, December 2021.

Grimmer, Justin, Eitan Hersh, Marc Meredith, Jonathan Mummolo, and Clayton Nall, "Obstacles to Estimating Voter ID Laws' Effect on Turnout," *Journal of Politics*, Vol. 80, No. 3, 2018.

Hajnal, Zoltan, Nazita Lajevardi, and Lindsay Nielson, "Voter Identification Laws and the Suppression of Minority Votes," *Journal of Politics*, Vol. 79, No. 2, 2017.

Hodgson, Quentin E., Jennifer Kavanagh, Anusree Garg, Edward W. Chan, and Christine Sovak, *Options for Ensuring Safe Elections: Preparing for Elections During a Pandemic*, RAND Corporation, RR-A112-10, 2020. As of May 18, 2023:
https://www.rand.org/pubs/research_reports/RRA112-10.html

Hood, M. V., III, and William Gillespie, "They Just Do Not Vote Like They Used To: A Methodology to Empirically Assess Election Fraud," *Social Science Quarterly*, Vol. 93, No. 1, 2012.

"In-Person Voting Really Did Accelerate COVID-19's Spread in America," *The Economist*, July 10, 2021.

Kaplan, Ethan, and Haishan Yuan, "Early Voting Laws, Voter Turnout, and Partisan Vote Composition: Evidence from Ohio," *American Economic Journal: Applied Economics*, Vol. 12, No. 1, 2020.

Kavanagh, Jennifer, Quentin E. Hodgson, C. Ben Gibson, and Samantha Cherney, *An Assessment of State Voting Processes: Preparing for Elections During a Pandemic*, RAND Corporation, RR-A112-8, 2020. As of March 22, 2022:
https://www.rand.org/pubs/research_reports/RRA112-8.html

Lai, Jonathan, "New Pennsylvania Absentee Ballot Rules Mean Early Voting for 2020 Election," *Inquirer*, January 14, 2020.

Manson, Steven, Jonathan Schroeder, David Van Riper, Tracy Kugler, and Steven Ruggles, IPUMS National Historical Geographic Information System, database, Version 16.0, 2021. As of May 18, 2023:
https://www.ipums.org/projects/ipums-nhgis/d050.v16.0

Mitchell, Amy, Mark Jurkowitz, J. Baxter Oliphant, and Elisa Shearer, "1. Legitimacy of Voting by Mail Politicized, Leaving Americans Divided," Pew Research Center, September 16, 2020. As of March 22, 2022:
https://www.pewresearch.org/journalism/2020/09/16/legitimacy-of-voting-by-mail-politicized-leaving-americans-divided/

National Conference of State Legislatures, "Same Day Voter Registration," webpage, September 20, 2021. As of March 22, 2022:
https://www.ncsl.org/research/elections-and-campaigns/same-day-registration.aspx

O'Dea, Colleen, "NJ Moves to Strengthen November's Mail-In Election," *NJ Spotlight News*, August 28, 2020.

Pew Research Center, "Republicans, Democrats Move Even Further Apart in Coronavirus Concerns," June 25, 2020a. As of March 22, 2022:
https://www.pewresearch.org/politics/2020/06/25/republicans-democrats-move-even-further-apart-in-coronavirus-concerns/

Pew Research Center, "3. The Voting Experience in 2020," November 20, 2020b. As of March 22, 2022:
https://www.pewresearch.org/politics/2020/11/20/the-voting-experience-in-2020/

Quealy, Kevin and Alicia Parlapiano, "Election Day Voting in 2020 Took Longer in America's Poorest Neighborhoods," *New York Times*, January 4, 2021.

Riker, William H., and Peter C. Ordeshook, "A Theory of the Calculus of Voting," *American Political Science Review*, Vol. 62, No. 1, 1968.

Schraufnagel, Scot, Michael J. Pomante, and Quan Li, "Cost of Voting in American States: 2022," *Election Law Journal: Rules, Politics, and Policy*, Vol. 21 No. 3, 2022.

Stewart, Charles, III, *How We Voted in 2020: A Topical Look at the Survey of the Performance of American Elections*, MIT Election Data + Science Lab, December 15, 2020. As of March 22, 2022:
http://electionlab.mit.edu/sites/default/files/2021-03/HowWeVotedIn2020-March2021.pdf

Tyson, Alec, "Republicans Remain Far Less Likely Than Democrats to View COVID-19 as a Major Threat to Public Health," Pew Research Center, July 22, 2020. As of March 22, 2022:
https://www.pewresearch.org/fact-tank/2020/07/22/republicans-remain-far-less-likely-than-democrats-to-view-COVID-19-as-a-major-threat-to-public-health/

Weil, Matthew, Charles Stewart, III, Tim Harper, Christopher Thomas, Erin Barry, Sarah Kline, and Owen Minott, "The 2018 Voting Experience: Polling Place Lines," *Bipartisan Policy Center*, November 4, 2019.

Williams, Corey, "Why Blacks Distrust Voting by Mail," *Columbus Dispatch*, August 2, 2020.

Wines, Michael, "COVID-19 Changed How We Vote. It Could Also Change Who Votes," *New York Times*, June 14, 2020.

Wu, Jennifer, Chenoa Yorgason, Hanna Folsz, Cassandra Handan-Nader, Andrew Myers, Tobias Nowacki, Daniel M. Thompson, Jesse Yoder, and Andrew B. Hall, "Are Dead People Voting By Mail? Evidence From Washington State Administrative Records," *Democracy & Polarization*, Stanford University, 2020.

Yoder, Jesse, Cassandra Handan-Nader, Andrew Myers, Tobias Nowacki, Daniel M. Thompson, Jennifer A. Wu, Chenoa Yorgason, and Andrew B. Hall, "How Did Absentee Voting Affect the 2020 U.S. Election?" *Science Advances*, Vol. 7, No. 52, 2021.